INTRODUCTION TO HEALTH SCIENCES LIBRARIANSHIP

Recent Titles in
The Greenwood Library Management Collection

Library Records: A Retention and Confidentiality Guide
Shirley A. Wiegand

Managing Performing Arts Collections in Academic and Public Libraries
Carolyn A. Sheehy, editor

Video Collection Development in Multi-type Libraries: A Handbook
Gary P. Handman, editor

A Library Manager's Guide to the Physical Processing of Nonprint Materials
Karen C. Driessen and Sheila A. Smyth

The Challenge and Practice of Academic Accreditation: A Sourcebook for Library Administrators
Edward D. Garten, editor

Information Services for People with Developmental Disabilities
Linda Lucas Walling and Marilyn M. Irwin, editors

Public Library Planning: Case Studies for Management
Brett Sutton

Video Acquisitions and Cataloging: A Handbook
James C. Scholtz

Introducing and Managing Academic Library Automation Projects
John W. Head and Gerard B. McCabe, editors

The National Electronic Library: A Guide to the Future for Library Managers
Gary M. Pitkin, editor

Strategic Management for Public Libraries: A Handbook
Robert M. Hayes and Virginia A. Walter

Managing Business Collections in Libraries
Carolyn A. Sheehy, editor

Introduction to Health Sciences Librarianship

A MANAGEMENT HANDBOOK

Frank R. Kellerman

THE GREENWOOD LIBRARY MANAGEMENT COLLECTION
Gerard B. McCabe, Series Adviser

GREENWOOD PRESS
Westport, Connecticut • London

Library of Congress Cataloging-in-Publication Data

Kellerman, Frank R.
Introduction to health sciences librarianship : a management handbook / Frank R. Kellerman.
p. cm.—(The Greenwood library management collection, ISSN 0894–2986)
Includes bibliographical references and index.
ISBN 0–313–29761–4 (alk. paper)
1. Medical libraries—United States. I. Title. II. Series.
Z675.M4K44 1997
026.61—dc20 96–8427

British Library Cataloguing in Publication Data is available.

Library of Congress Catalog Card Number: 96–8427
ISBN: 0–313–29761–4
ISSN: 0894–2986

First published in 1997

Greenwood Press, 88 Post Road West, Westport, CT 06881
An imprint of Greenwood Publishing Group, Inc.

Printed in the United States of America

The paper used in this book complies with the Permanent Paper Standard issued by the National Information Standards Organization (Z39.48–1984).

10 9 8 7 6 5 4 3 2

To Brook, Grant, Eva,
Sophie, and Walter

Contents

Preface

Health sciences librarianship today demands a balance among computer files, human ingenuity, and print sources. Thanks to computerization and telecommunications, librarians can do much more now than just a few years ago. With access to information at the heart of a library's purpose, those tools have opened up new worlds to us. We cannot yet, however, depend altogether on a fully computerized, virtual library. Admittedly, in science, the conventional wisdom has long assumed that books are out of date when published. However, in biomedicine we still need and use books as well as other paper resources. We need both to develop new ways of finding and utilizing information and to use many of our traditional skills. Although the field is now more interesting than ever, perhaps it would have been easier to come into health sciences librarianship ten or twenty years ago. The librarian's objective remains the same—the need to get the right information to the health professionals when they need it. The many more sources available now to meet that goal enable us to do a better and more thorough job. This also means a lot more for us to learn. This book is a start. It is an introduction to an exciting field.

An effort will be made here (not always successfully) to avoid some of the usual hyperbole (e.g., ''explosive'' growth of the literature; ''proliferation'' of journals; and the Internet as the ''superhighway''). However, it would be difficult for anyone to open a newspaper or hear a radio or television news program and not be presented with an announcement relating to a biomedical discovery. Some publications are specifically devoted to bringing the highlights of medicine to the public's attention. The *Harvard Health Letter* is an example, and it even annually ranks the top ten advances in medicine. The findings reported on radio and television may turn out to be valid and useful, or they may not. A gene has been identified that can be linked to many cases of colon cancer. A combination of drugs may have potential in treating AIDS. Cardiovascular disease may be sharply reduced by adhering to a specific diet and exercise regimen. Breast cancer diagnostic tools are safe and accurate, or later that same day from a different authority, they are unsafe and inaccurate. The dramatic accounts make good news stories. The subject of medicine is not obscure and is not limited in interest to a handful of scientists with their investigations. Our personal health is of immediate interest to all of us. As individuals, we are exposed to health information and health advice daily. It is no surprise to hear that there is a lot of health information available. The point is that news reports present a small fraction of the studies of thousands of scientists. It is not a simple matter, therefore, for a practicing physician or a researcher to find out about everything that will be of importance to his or her patients or research. Here is where the medical librarian enters the picture, finding the right information. Parenthetically, although "medical" and "health sciences" are not synonymous, the terms "medical librarian" and "health sciences librarian" are used interchangeably in this book, as they often are in the field.

The journal literature stubbornly retains its preeminence in medicine as the medium for information. Chapter 1 examines the roles that the journal plays as well as the great proportion of our budgets it consumes. Information retrieval is the reason for librarianship, and Chapters 2 and 3 focus on techniques of searching the journal literature. We rely on the traditional abstracting and indexing tools whether in print or computer. (Even in the 1990s, there are still two good reasons for examining the paper indexes. The computer version is based on their structure, and the older material, pre-1960s, is still in paper.) Recent developments help us find not just the relevant information but also the pertinent (i.e., useable). Whereas in the past we would have merely supplied the clinician with a list of articles on the topic of the patient's disease, today we can often tailor the information we deliver so that it is suitable for the doctor to use directly in treatment.

Chapters 4 and 5 introduce you to the selection and organization of health sciences books and then to reference tools and services. When you need to refer to a comprehensive collection, look for *Current Practice in Health Sciences Librarianship* (Bunting 1994–), the eight-volume set under development by the Medical Library Association. This is the successor to *Handbook of Medical Library Practice* (Darling 1982–88), which ended in a fourth edition. Also, Roper and Boorkman (1994) have updated their excellent work on reference sources. The key reference for librarians in hospitals has been *Hospital Library Management* (Bradley 1983). There are plans for a new edition. A fairly recent issue of *Library Trends* (Dalrymple 1993) is devoted to developments in our field. Consult, too, the journal literature of the profession, especially the *Bulletin of the Medical Library Association*, which you will see cited throughout this book, and also *Medical Reference Services Quarterly*.

Chapter 6 is ''Computerization of Biomedical Information.'' This chapter does more than cite books and journals and indexes and catalogs. It attempts to portray the variety of medical information becoming available. Information on the gene linked to colon cancer, for example, can be found in the molecular biology databanks. On the clinical side, physicians may be aided in their decision making by expert system programs that house algorithms for diagnoses. Only a few snapshots of the developments in computerized information can be presented here. There is so much happening on the Internet, as well as in-house applications. For more information beyond Chapter 6 on these advances, go to the primary literature—the biomedical literature. This is part of the excitement and the importance, too, of the field of health sciences librarianship. Biomedicine is dynamic, and you have the keys to its information at your fingertips.

What else makes health sciences librarianship different? Our environments do. Chapter 7 covers the library settings (hospital, medical school, and research institute), history (through our national library), networks (organizational and electronic), professional associations and organizations (library and biomedical), and economics (micro and macro). Our health is of great interest not only to us as individuals. The cost of our health care has been increasingly captivating to our organizations (e.g., hospitals) and to society (taxpayers). The economic dimensions and pressures as well as all the other ''environments'' affect how we are doing our jobs. We need this information to run our libraries.

Let us turn now to our literature. Our storehouse of information continues to be dominated by paper—the paper journal. Moving to electronic formats will certainly make a big difference to our patrons and to us. However, many features and problems will carry over from paper. You will need to understand the varied issues presented by the biomedical journal, which therefore deserves an in-depth examination.

Abbreviations and Acronyms

AAAS	American Association for the Advancement of Science
AAHSLD	Association of Academic Health Sciences Library Directors
ABMS	American Board of Medical Specialties
AHA	American Hospital Association
AHCPR	Agency for Health Care Policy Research
AHIMA	American Health Information Management Association
AIM	*Abridged Index Medicus*
AIM/TWX	*Abridged Index Medicus*/Teletypewriter Exchange
ALA	American Library Association
AMA	American Medical Association
AMRA	American Medical Records Association
AVLINE	Audiovisuals Online
BA	*Biological Abstracts*
BA/RRM	*Biological Abstracts/Reports, Reviews, Meetings*
BIOSIS	BioSciences Information Service
BLAB	Biomedical Library Acquisitions Bulletin
BLAST	Basic Local Alignment Search Tool
BRS	Bibliographic Retrieval Services
CA	*Chemical Abstracts*

CANCERLIT	Cancer Literature
CAS	*Chemical Abstracts* Service
CASSI	*Chemical Abstracts Service Source Index*
CATLINE	Catalog Online
CC	*Current Contents*
CDC	Centers for Disease Control
CINAHL	*Cumulative Index to Nursing and Allied Health Literature*
CIP	Cataloging in Publication
CQI/TQM	Continuous Quality Improvement/Total Quality Management
CRISP	Computer Retrieval of Information on Scientific Projects
dh	Diet Therapy (subheading)
DNA	Deoxyribonucleic Acid
DRG	Diagnostic Related Group
dt	Drug Therapy (subheading)
ELHILL	The MEDLARS searching software named after Senator Lister Hill
EM	*Excerpta Medica*
EMBASE	*Excerpta Medica* Database
EXP	Explode or Explosion
FASEB	Federation of American Societies for Experimental Biology
FDA	Food and Drug Administration
FREIDA	Fellowship and Residency Electronic Interactive Database Access
GALEN	Generalized Architecture for Languages, Encyclopedias, and Nomenclatures
GDB	Genome Data Base
GDP	Gross Domestic Product
GNP	Gross National Product
GPEP	General Professional Education of the Physician
GRACE	Graphic Arts Composing Equipment
HANES	(National) Health and Nutrition Examination Survey
HCFA	Health Care Financing Administration
HSTAR	Health Services/Technology Assessment Research
HSTAT	Health Services/Technology Assessment Text
IAIMS	Integrated Academic (or Advanced) Information Management System
IDL	*Index to Dental Literature*
IM	*Index Medicus*
INI	*International Nursing Index*
IPA	*International Pharmaceutical Abstracts*
JAMA	*Journal of the American Medical Association*

JCAHO	Joint Commission on Accreditation of Healthcare Organizations
JCR	*Journal Citation Reports*
KWIC	Key Word in Context
KWOC	Key Word Out of Context
LC	Library of Congress
MARC	Machine Readable Cataloging
MedIndEx	Medical Indexing Expert (System)
MEDLARS	Medical Literature Analysis and Retrieval System
MEDLINE	MEDLARS Online
MeSH	*Medical Subject Headings*
MH	MeSH Heading
MHF	MeSH Heading Fragment
MLA	Medical Library Association
MLAA	Medical Library Assistance Act
MLANET	Medical Library Association Network
NBR	Neighbor
NCLEX-RN	National Council Licensure Examination for Registered Nurses
NHANES	National Health and Nutrition Examination Survey
NIH	National Institutes of Health
NIM	Non *Index Medicus*
NLM	National Library of Medicine
NN/LM	National Network of Libraries of Medicine
NTIS	National Technical Information Service
OCLC	Online Computer Library Center (formerly Ohio College Library Center)
OJCCT	*Online Journal of Current Clinical Trials*
OMIM	Online Mendelian Inheritance in Man
OPAC	Online Public Access Catalog
PA	*Psychological Abstracts*
PDQ	Physician Data Query
PDR	*Physicians Desk Reference*
PsycINFO	*Psychological Abstracts* Information Services
PX	Pre-Explode or Pre-Explosion
QA	Quality Assurance
QCIM	*Quarterly Cumulative Index Medicus*
RLIN	Research Libraries Information Network
RMLP	Regional Medical Library Program
SAIL	System for Automated Interlibrary Loan

SCI	*Science Citation Index*
SDC	System Development Corporation
SERHOLD	Serials Holdings
SERLINE	Serials Online
SPEC	Specialty
SPIN	Sponsored Programs Information Network
su	Surgery (subheading)
SUNY	State University of New York
TF	Title Field
th	Therapy (subheading)
TOXNET	Toxicology Data Network
TQM	Total Quality Management
TW	Text Word
UCMP	Union Catalog of Medical Periodicals
UMLS	Unified Medical Language System
URL	Uniform Resource Locator
USDA	United States Department of Agriculture
USP	United States Pharmacopeia
VNS	Virtual Notebook System
WIN	Westlaw Is Natural
WONDER	Wide-ranging Online Data for Epidemiologic Research

INTRODUCTION TO HEALTH SCIENCES LIBRARIANSHIP

1

The Biomedical Journal

INTRODUCTION

Imagine your physician treating you for a medical condition he or she does not fully understand. Visualize your physician running through his or her mind the experiences he or she has had with the symptoms you are presenting. Think of your doctor analyzing your case and needing more information on what treatment(s) would be best for you. You may not have to think too hard or long on these scenarios. This could very well have happened to you and your doctor more than once. Many times patients do not fit into textbook solutions. Everyone knows that physicians cannot rely solely on the medical textbooks they used in school. They cannot even rely totally on the most current editions of those authoritative publications. It may be the case that there is no accepted remedy that works very well for your ailment. It may be the case that research has been developing no promising treatments. Or it may be that your doctor is unaware of either the research going on or even the accepted treatment for that disease. Your doctor cannot know everything that is going on in medicine on all diseases. He or she always needs more up-to-date information. This is what, seemingly, the journal literature can do. In general, the role of the health sciences librarian is to provide the health care professionals with the information they need. This involves the full range of skills and background we develop from acquiring to organizing to retrieving information in many formats residing in and outside our libraries. As with the doctor, we also need to keep learning how to do our job better. Often today, however, our role specifically entails finding the right journal articles that answer the question the doctor or researcher or nurse or hospital administrator or other health care professional has. In order for you to deliver that service, you need a thorough understanding of the journal literature and the many issues involved with it. An examination of the biomedical journal is a fitting place to start.

HISTORY

The role of and the problems with the scientific journal have been argued about for years. It continues to be a topic of debate in the literature of library science and the biomedical and physical sciences. The journal article seems like a perfect vehicle for scientific information. Science progresses by increments. A journal article typically addresses a narrow topic. Scientific communication places a premium on currency. Journal issues come out relatively fast—at least more quickly than books. However, there is a lot more to this story. The seventeenth century brought the start of the modern scientific journal. The first two were *Journal des Scavans* (1665) and *Philosophical Transactions of the Royal Society of London* (1666). Groups of individuals with common interests in science met together to report on their experiments and findings. Publication of the reports of the meetings provided a useful service to the members. By the nineteenth century, the journal was well established as the preeminent form of medical literature. Oliver Wendell Holmes, in 1881, put it this way:

> A library, to meet the need of our time, must take, and must spread out in a convenient form, a great array of periodicals. Our active practitioners read these by preference over almost everything else. Our specialists, more particularly, depend on the month's product, on the yearly crop of new facts, new suggestions, new contrivances, as much as the farmer on the annual yield of his acres. (Fye 1987, 453)

The medical literature at the turn of the century reported on cases, proposed cures, and offered random observations. To a greater extent in Europe than in the United States, scientific medical research was undertaken and the literature reported those findings. After the reform of medical education with the Flexner Report (1910) in the United States, opportunities for medical research became more abundant. Medical schools began to employ full-time teachers instead of relying totally on the part-time contributions of the practitioners. Emphasis was placed on research and publication of the research. The place where they published their research was in the medical journals. World War II and the succeeding years brought a great increase in funding for research. There were many more individuals doing research and writing for publication, so the growth of the biomedical literature continued. More and more journals came into being. The natural solution was specialization and subspecialization and the fragmentation of knowledge and the literature. Complaining over the impossibility of keeping up-to-date in a field has been a popular pastime. Quotations demonstrating this phenomenon give us an entertaining literary spin-off.

> In the beginning was the General Scientific Journal. And the General Scientific Journal begat the Specialty Journal, and the Specialty Journal begat the Subspecialty Journal. . . . And the scientific community saw that the journals were good, and they were fruitful and multiplied. So the National Journals (e.g., British, American, and Canadian) begat the Supranational Journals. . . . And the whole scientific literature became overweight, unreadable. . . . (Berry 1981, 400–401)

Durack (1978) elevated this discussion another step. In his article "The Weight of Medical Knowledge," the author is pictured smiling next to a scale weighing the one volume of the 1879 *Index Medicus* (IM) and weary next to the many volumes that made up the 1974 IM. A 1992 commentary suggests, "uses journal as a pillow during nights on call" (Bennett 1992, 920). Such jokes are entertaining and do reflect how many view the literature. The growth in the number of journals and journal articles is constantly written about, argued about, and moaned about.

SCIENTIFIC COMMUNICATION

Although librarians and scientists do complain about the thousands of biomedical journals, the growth can be seen as a not unreasonable development. The number of scientists at work has grown, too. "The peculiar immediacy of science, the recognition that so large a proportion of everything scientific that has ever occurred is happening now, within living memory. To put it another way, using any reasonable definition of a scientist, we can say that 80 to 90 percent of all the scientists that have ever lived are alive now" (Price 1986, 1). (It may be difficult to confirm that estimation by Price, but it sounds right.) The goal of science is to expand our knowledge. Each scientist, it may be argued, contributes a small bit of new knowledge. Scientists do not work in a vacuum. Isaac Newton's famous line still gives a picture of how the process is designed to work: "If I have seen further . . . it is by standing upon the shoulders of Giants" (Bartlett 1980, 313). Newton is acknowledging his debt to scientists who have come before. And so, too, the individual scientist now reads and acknowledges via citation in his paper the work of others. This is one reason for the scientific article and journal—to communicate with peers and successors.

In the biosciences, the emphasis is clearly on the recent information. Although the maintenance of the historical record is not a main concern for many biomedical libraries, we do have the obligation to preserve the record of science. (This issue might be brought more forcefully to our attention with electronic journals.) The journal performs the role of documenting the advances in scientific information, the steps along the way. This use is not limited to science historians. Biomedical researchers can use findings from the recent and more distant past. Results of yesteryear may be rediscovered and found to contain additional significance.

LEGITIMACY AND CLAIM TO THE IDEA

There is another role beyond keeping the record and facilitating scientific communication. After all, there are many ways to communicate. You can type up a note, photocopy it, and send it directly to all your colleagues in the Invisible College—those scholars all over the country or world who are working on the same specific topic you are. You can use your electronic correspondence or bulletin boards to quickly send your insights to the multitudes, far and wide. In this era, there are many more efficient ways to get out the word than submitting your formally worded article to a scientific journal. With journals, you hope your article will be accepted quickly, and you will be happy to see it published in a few months.

Why bother with this? It was good enough for the seventeenth century, but can we not do better? In fact, a lot of discussion continues on the electronic transfer of information. However, for now anyway, your revelation does not get the mark of legitimacy until it goes to a journal and passes the editorial and peer review process. You often see evidence of this. Scientists on occasion hold a press conference to trumpet their important discoveries directly to the public. Voices immediately rise up from the science community. Those findings cannot yet be accepted, they always say. The studies must be submitted to a peer review journal before any credence may be given. Why? Because the results must be made to stand up to formal scrutiny. Peer review is the way to measure the work, to see if it used proper scientific procedures. The results must be reproducible. Scientists need to do more than announce their conclusions. They must elaborate on the materials and methods. Although the reviewers will not often redo the experiment, they will have a lot to say from reading about the methodology. Evaluation of the methods will determine if the results and conclusions are warranted. This is the ethic of the scientist, the ingrained understanding. Parenthetically, the periodical that is designed to poke fun at science is called the *Journal of Irreproducible Results.* (Search under the Library of Congress Subject Heading "Science—Humor—Periodicals." You will find this, but not too many others.)

STRUCTURE OF THE SCIENTIFIC ARTICLE

The scientist writes an article describing the experiment and submits it to a journal. The form of the research article is prescribed. The title is often lengthy and should be informative. Clever but uninformative titles are not acceptable. Usually an abstract or summary of the research follows the title. The sections of the paper appear in this order: introduction, materials and methods, results, and summary and conclusions. The scientist began the project with a hypothesis.

In the introduction, he or she can note the state of knowledge up to the present in order to give background information to the reader and demonstrate how the proposed hypothesis fits in. The materials and methods section describes how the experiment was conducted. In what state of health and disease were the patients in the study? How many of them were there? How many test animals were there? Were they legitimate models of that disease? What dose did they get? Did they receive it orally or intravenously? And so forth. Then in the results section the scientist gives the findings that came out of the experiment. Tables of laboratory results are presented. Changes in symptoms are reported. In the summary and conclusions, the author can then tell the reader what this bit of new knowledge means and what it portends for future research and health care.

Here is an example of how parts of a research project may go into an article. Dr. Wolff investigated the use of Drug K to treat asthma. The introduction describes current treatments for asthma, the uses of Drug K, and Dr. Wolff's hypothesis—Drug K is useful for treating asthma. In the materials and methods section, Dr. Wolff tells how he did a double blind study. For the next thirty asthma patients, he gives either Drug K or a placebo. The placebo looks the same as Drug K but has no therapeutic ingredients. The patients do not know which of them got Drug K, and Dr. Wolff does not know which received Drug K. That is the meaning of the term "double blind." Not all studies are done in this manner. The results section carries the laboratory data and clinical observations. Ten of the fifteen who took Drug K improved, whereas three of those with the placebo improved. In the conclusion, Dr. Wolff says that Drug K has utility in the treatment of asthma. The next step he plans is the use of larger doses. This stage of the research is finished and written up in the format of a journal article. Now Dr. Wolff sends off his manuscript to a journal.

PEER REVIEW

As we have heard, there are many journals in each field. Scientists would like their work published in the most prestigious journal in their field. In choosing the journal, the first requirement is that it be peer reviewed. Once the editor of the journal reads the article, he or she determines if it fits the scope of the journal. If the paper fits and the editor feels that it may have merit, he or she will send copies of the article to reviewers. Another name for a reviewer is referee. Reviewers are other scientists in the same specialty as Dr. Wolff. They are asked to give their expert opinion on the worthiness of Dr. Wolff's paper. Theoretically, the reviewers do not know who wrote the article and Dr. Wolff does not know who is reviewing his article. Because of the narrowness of fields—those subspecialties—and those Invisible Colleges, the identity of the other party can often be guessed. How are the reviewers able to evaluate the article? They can speak to the importance of the project and determine how it fits in with the rest of the research. Although they usually cannot repeat the experiment, they can evaluate the methodology. In this case, they might say that fifteen patients taking Drug K is not enough to be meaningful. They may feel that with such small numbers, extrapolation to a larger population is not called for. They may want to hear more about the previous conditions of the patients. The reviewers may find small problems or large problems with a study. The reviewers send their comments to the editor.

The editor then decides whether to publish Dr. Wolff's paper. The next question is, How does the editor decide? Is it a simple matter of majority rule? If two referees say the paper is sound and one referee says that it should be rejected, does the editor go ahead and publish it? For that matter, if all the referees say a study is worthless, does the editor always reject it? No. The power is in the editor's hands. In fact, the process has been fairly well hidden, and the power that the editor wields is an important issue to those wishing to get published. Concerns and problems were aired and addressed in two special issues of *JAMA* (Guarding the Guardians 1990; International Congress on Peer Review 1994). In recent years, some journals have taken pains to describe their practices explicitly. For instance, they may reveal the number of papers submitted to them, their rejection rate, the number of referees used per paper, the input of assistant editors, and the number of papers rejected prior to the review process. There is often another outcome besides outright acceptance or rejection. Comments from the editor and the referees are passed along to the author with suggestions on how to strengthen the paper and the research. The paper can then be resubmitted with a high likelihood of acceptance.

Robert Lucky of Bell Laboratories has this, perhaps partly humorous, assessment:

> [T]he reviewer has received the paper from the editor with a request for an opinion. As befits the dignity attached to rendering such a judgment, the reviewer first hurriedly turns to the back of the paper to see if he himself has been referenced. Probably he has been, since this is how the editor generally selects reviewers, but heaven help the author if he has neglected to reference such important work that might have been published by the reviewer. (Lucky 1989, 144)

From most of this description, you might see why scientists find difficulty with periodic declarations via press conferences and news releases. If a researcher does an experiment, gets his results, comes to conclusions, and then tells the world, it is his voice alone. If, on the other hand, the scientist goes through the peer review process, the findings have a legitimacy placed upon them by the science community. It should not be assumed that the study was well done or the results accurate or the conclusions warranted. It also does not mean that everyone agrees with what the author said in the paper. However, after publication, the study does take its place among the millions of other articles and small steps in scientific progress.

A SCIENTIST'S CAREER AND ITS IMPACT ON THE JOURNAL

Science is a cooperative endeavor. Each researcher adds a small piece of knowledge to the ever-growing accumulation of scientific truths. Along with cooperation, science is a very competitive enterprise. Individuals compete for funds to do the research. They compete for publication in the prestigious journals. They also compete for promotion, tenure, and professional awards. Scientists compete for promotion and standing in their field by demonstrating a record of accomplishment. How do they prove their worth? In what manner do they show that they are good scientists and are making substantial contributions to science? All they need to do is pull out their curriculum vitae and show their list of journal articles.

This method of validating credentials affects the growth of the literature. A long list of articles is prima facie evidence of a productive career. It means that a lot of articles will be submitted to journals for publication. It also means, therefore, that new journals will keep cropping up to receive the abundance of the larger and larger numbers of scientists. Existing journals will often grow. Quarterlies will become bimonthlies. Bimonthlies will become monthlies. Monthlies will become semimonthlies.

It is correct to contend that the journal's role is scientific communication. A hypothesis receives legitimacy by publication, and the message is widely distributed. The scientist receives the credit. Credits may be tabulated, unfortunately, by counting the number of papers. This leads to two other practices. Although there is usually a principal investigator for an experiment, more than one person typically is involved. This makes sense. Individuals bring different expertise to the parts of the project. However, it is not uncommon to have five or ten or fifteen scientists as co-authors of a journal article. Remember, these articles are often five to ten pages in length, and there are cases of 40, 50, and more authors' names on a paper. Thelma Charen of the National Library of Medicine's Indexing Section notes the extreme of this phenomenon. In the decision to limit the number of names from an article to the first ten for the IM author index, she noted the following: "A story which searchers think is apocryphal concerns an article in a Japanese journal with over 100 authors. It is not apocryphal. . . . One day in 1986 I encountered what I consider the new Heavyweight Champion of Japanese Authorship: an article submitted by 193 authors" (Charen 1988, 14). Since that time, new "records" have been set. A large clinical trial by 972 co-authors appeared in the *New England Journal of Medicine* (McDonald 1995). Why does this happen? The more papers that you have on your curriculum vitae, the more productive you are. In the case from Japan, it appears that the name of each person at the sponsoring institutions was included.

Okay, you say, this is not fooling anybody. Fifty people cannot have made meaningful contributions to a five-page paper. Probably the first author listed is the real investigator. From that attitude, another pernicious practice has evolved. Let's say there is a study with five authors. A convenient solution is to segment the work. The authors may submit five different articles to parallel the progress along the way of the study. Rotating each of the five authors to the first author's spot in one article makes everybody happy. Each author can claim a lot of credit. The foregoing presumed a structured order to the listing of authors; that is, the first name on the paper was that of the person most responsible. Although no universal prescription exists, now and then guidelines are proposed to regulate who should and should not be included as authors and how their names should be ordered in the paper (Riesenberg and Lundberg 1990).

By its nature, science is a fragmented business. However, the foregoing practice needlessly adds to the fragmentation. Using the "least publishable unit" does not help science and it does not help the library's growing serials budget. What can be done? A few years ago, Harvard University Medical School devised an interesting approach (Harvard Guidelines 1989). When scientists apply for promotion, they submit a list of their publications. This is certainly not new. What the guidelines proposed was a requirement of an upper limit instead of a lower limit on what could be submitted. If five articles are the limit for a specific position in the medical school, the scientist better make sure that those five are high-quality, complete articles and that he or she is a major contributor to them.

HANDLING THE BIOMEDICAL LITERATURE

We have just discussed the supply side, as it were, of scientific literature, which needs to be written to communicate, to legitimize one's idea, and to advance one's own career. However, what is the demand? Who wants to read it? Communication implies two parties, at least—one sending and one receiving. There must be a party on the receiving end for successful communication. The difficulty of keeping up on everything relevant to the scientist's work has been noted. This is not a theoretical problem. Are people actually reading the literature? Physicians have the same concern. With so much happening, even in their subspecialty, how can they know what is known? People read at about the same rate as they did when there were one-tenth as many journals and one-one-hundreth as many journals. Perhaps they might just read the summaries or abstracts—and whether to do so may very well be worth examining—but a cautionary note is needed. Remember, an experiment is no better than its methodology. Scientists and clinicians must not accept a finding just because it is in print. They need to use their critical skills to evaluate the studies.

From the librarian's point of view, we can take some consolation in Bradford's Law (also known as Bradford's Law of Scattering or the Bradford Distribution). Samuel Bradford (1934) was very concerned in the 1930s that scientists and engineers were missing important information because the abstracting and indexing services could not include every journal that might have articles of possible relevance. He investigated further and found that articles on a specific topic tended to cluster in a relatively small number of journals. Articles were not scattered evenly throughout the many journals of a discipline. He ranked journals by the number of articles that they had on that topic. For this, ranking was based solely on quantity. A few journals had many articles on the topic, a larger number of journals had a few articles each on the topic, and many journals had just one article on that topic. A reader or library could be fairly confident in covering the topic to a great extent, but not exhaustively, by reading or collecting a relatively few journals.

Take this contrived example. We want to know how the literature on malaria is scattered throughout the biomedical journals. After a thorough search of the literature, we ranked the journals by how productive they were (i.e., the top journal had the largest number of articles on malaria). We continued on down until we listed all the journals that had just one article on malaria. Here is a summary of the findings. A total of 9,000 articles were found on malaria. The top ten journals had a total of 3,000 articles. How many journals, going down through the list of productivity, would it take to include about 3,000 more articles? You count down the list and find that it takes 50 more journals to get those next 3,000 articles. How many more journals does it take to collect all the rest—the 3,000 remaining articles? You meticulously go through the list and find that it takes 250 additional journals to get the last 3,000 articles. Here is a summary in tabular form.

Group	Number of Articles	Number of Journals
1	3,000	10
2	3,000	50
3	3,000	250

This example was set up in order to fit Bradford's scheme neatly. The number of journals in the groups have the ratios that Bradford postulated—1 : n : n times n. In our example, n = 5. There are five times the number of journals in group 2 than in group 1; five times the number in group 3 than in group 2.

For Bradford's studies, the number of journals considered was modest. What about today, sixty years later? The number of journals is much larger. Bradford's Law of Scattering works to different degrees in various fields, but it does seem to work. And as more and more people get involved in science, questions of inquiry become more and more narrow. Specialties and subspecialties and sub-subspecialties develop. That may enable the physician to keep up with the bulk of a narrow subspecialty by reading a relatively small number of journals. How do they find the rest of the literature when they need it? They will want or need to find out about studies in related areas. It will be difficult to find out about those other studies if they just scan their core journals. An answer from librarians is the abstracting and indexing services, which will be discussed in the next chapter.

HIGH-QUALITY JOURNALS, POWER, AND THE INGELFINGER RULE

Bradford was measuring quantity only. Size is, certainly, not the only or most important factor. All scientists will readily admit that not all journals covering a topic are equal. Some consistently publish studies of high quality and importance. Some are widely known and prestigious. Scientists want to publish in prestigious journals and know which ones those are. Arnold Relman (1981) was the editor of the prominent *New England Journal of Medicine*. His point of view is this: Read the good journals. Do not worry about what is in the others. The important advances will be in the good journals. The good journals have high rejection rates. Papers that are rejected by the *New England Journal of Medicine* and other good journals will be resubmitted to journals of lesser renown and will eventually get published somewhere. As librarians, how do we feel about this? To a certain extent, we follow this line of reasoning in our purchasing decisions. We try to buy the best journals in the subject fields of interest to our patrons. Yet this leaves tremendous power in the hands of a relatively few editors. The implications of disregarding such a large chunk of the literature are great. It is our duty as librarians to inform our clientele about the information that is out there. On the other hand, do we need to inundate our patrons? Can we help them get the high-quality material? There remains the problem of an underuse of the literature by physicians. Nor are the advances of research being brought to physicians in a timely manner. We will get back to this in Chapter 5.

The preface noted the newsworthiness of medical information. Many of the items carried in the daily newspapers and in the electronic media come directly from the reports of a few medical journals. *JAMA—The Journal of the American Medical Association* and the *New England Journal of Medicine*, both weekly publications, are favorites for news stories. The appearance of an article in one of these peer-reviewed publications gives the information a level of legitimacy. As soon as an issue of the *New England Journal of Medicine* is made available to the news media, articles are summarized for the lay audience and appear in the newspaper and on television and radio. Actually, that is not quite correct. The *New England Journal of Medicine* has an agreement with the news media and has effectively set an embargo. The journal will release the contents to the press early in the week, but the press cannot report on the information until the middle of the week, when the journal's subscribers (physicians, among others) have received their copy. The information has been considered so newsworthy that newspapers and television stations would immediately report it to the public, before the professionals (physicians) had a chance to see the journal and therefore evaluate the article in full. Patients would call up their doctors to ask them about the media report, and the doctors would have no more information than the lay-level summary. Also partly designed for this reason is the Ingelfinger Rule, named for a former editor of that journal (Angell and Kassirer 1991).

This rule stipulates that the *New England Journal of Medicine* will not publish an article if its substance has already been announced or published elsewhere. This shows that not all of these thousands of publications are unread and destined only to collect dust.

Is this a satisfactory system for disseminating medical information? Should so much power be in the hands of the editors? This issue may be linked with the peer review situation, too. We are concerned with the subject of health and disease. In other words, these actually are life and death matters. What happens when a discovery is made that is of great consequence, one that would help thousands of people? Keeping the news out of the newspaper is just a matter of a few days. However, the wait for the completion of the peer review procedure may take months. Just how long is it legitimate to wait for the unveiling of the news? The editors say that they will expedite information that is of timely and critical importance. The reasoned review process must have a chance, they maintain, in order to weed out the flawed studies. The National Library of Medicine (NLM) took a step to address this problem. In January 1991, NLM announced a plan to handle urgent findings. ''Occasionally information learned while the [clinical] trial is in progress or at its conclusion is of such significance that if it were known and implemented by health care providers, the morbidity and mortality of the public would be reduced. . . . NLM is developing a program whereby users of the MEDLARS system will be informed electronically of clinical alerts'' (Colaianni 1991).

Although this type of mechanism can prove very useful, we should not totally forget the editors' warnings. To reach beyond biomedicine, consider the example of cold fusion. In 1989, the world heard of cold fusion directly from the two investigators, Martin Fleischmann and Stanley Pons, at a press conference and through the newspaper accounts of that announcement. The whole world was excited at the idea of cold fusion and the prospect of cheap energy. The details, the methods and materials, were not specified. Many scientists attempted to produce the results claimed by the two chemists from Utah. So far it has not been done. ''Fleischmann and Pons claim much better reproducibility. But until they divulge their method and results, kept secret so as not to invalidate patent applications, and tell the rest of us how to do it, it will remain difficult to counter the widespread rejection, which is often given to phenomena that cannot be reproduced at will by independent colleagues'' (Bockris 1991, 51). Even now it has not been reproduced. Perhaps it will someday. This was a convincing case of the role of peer review and scientific oversight.

SELECTION OF JOURNALS

There comes a time when you need to move beyond the philosophizing about the history and social implications of the biomedical journal. You need to decide which journals to buy for your collection. First, it should be acknowledged, there is a real difference between ordering a book and starting a journal subscription. The book is ordered, it arrives, you pay for it and hope to use it well. You order the journal and pay for it, and somewhat later the issues start to come in. You may even get additional bills for the time period of the journal you had thought that you had already paid for. Journals are meant to continue on into the indefinite future. The subscription is ongoing. Typically, subscriptions are renewed annually. You may choose to stop the subscription at that time. As a matter of fact, however, factors do inhibit this rational pattern of behavior (e.g., wanting to continue a nice run of years of a journal title, and maybe experiencing some inertia, too). Once the journal has been ordered and received, it will most likely be continued year after year. Libraries and serials librarians do not often take the zero-based budget approach, wherein you would evaluate your patrons' needs and your collection annually. Then, based on that information, you would select journals to be ordered that year. The more common incentive to evaluate your journal holdings is a budget problem and the need to cancel some titles. A few journals are then targeted for cancellation. This may not be the ideal way to oversee your collection, but it is often the practice. Realistically, therefore, you need to view selection of journals as a long-term investment. It will usually be an expensive, long-term investment. As is true with most library collections, in the eras of plenty as well as the tight times, you cannot get everything you want or need. There are a number of criteria that you can use to determine which journals should be in your collection.

INSTITUTIONAL SPECIALIZATION

The first step is to thoroughly examine the subjects with which your institution and your patrons are involved. In a health sciences library the range of subjects collected is different from a general collection. Going a step further, the institution that is served by a health sciences library usually has areas of relative strength within the health sciences. Your hospital may specialize in cancer therapy. Your organization may be doing materials research for the development of artificial organs. You may be supporting a nurse practitioner program. Your collection may be used by a dental school. In other words, the particular needs of your clientele will tell you what subject areas need to be covered. The journal collection is concentrated in those areas. The collection development policy, which will be discussed in Chapter 4, reflects the needs of the institution. After you have matched your collection against the needs of the institution and your patrons, you may go on to other criteria.

PATRON REQUESTS

Numerous suggestions for purchases will come from your patrons themselves. These requests are important. Your patrons are the people who will be using the material, and they will know what they need. You most likely will not be able to buy everything that all patrons request. Therefore, it is up to you to oversee the whole collection and not buy everything for one or two vocal patrons and little for others. If some needs are transitory, it may be better to utilize interlibrary loan or other means. Frequently, patrons request brand-new journals. In fact, many times the journal has not yet come out. On the basis of the editorial board, your scientists tell you, ''They are the leaders in my field and the papers in this journal will be of high quality.'' Another phenomenon is that editorial boards change. Sometimes there is a mass defection from a journal, and the publication you are left with is the same in name only. The board left over some dispute, and the members have established a new journal to publish papers it would have had in the old journal. It would certainly be appropriate to look into this further. A subscription to the new title and a cancellation of the old may be in order. The needs of your patrons are not static, either, and you need to monitor them through time.

CITATION OF THE LITERATURE

We saw earlier in the chapter that Isaac Newton explained in a magnanimous moment his contributions to science by acknowledging those who came before him: he said that he had stood on the shoulders of giants. The journal literature is supposed to convey the incremental gains brought by the individual articles. Each article in the journal has references to earlier works. Earlier articles often cited by the succeeding literature thus seem to be making useful contributions. The SCI (*Science Citation Index*) tracks journal articles that have been cited. (Chapter 2 includes a more complete discussion of SCI.) Journals that contain many cited articles seem to be well-used publications. Scientists are reading those journals and building upon that information. You may want to consider this in judging journals. Doing so is somewhat more sophisticated than making the assumption that Bradford made about journals. He ranked journals by a productivity solely based on the number of articles published on topics. The *Science Citation Index* demonstrates a different scheme of weighting to individual articles. Each article is rated by the number of times it is cited. The weighting for a journal as a whole is the ''Impact Factor,'' ''a measure of the frequency with which the 'average article' in a journal has been cited in a particular year'' (Garfield 1989, 10A). Here is a simple and fictitious example. The *Journal of Clinical Medicine*, let's say, published 250 articles over a time period. In that time period, journal articles in the thousands of journals SCI indexes referenced articles that appeared in the *Journal of Clinical Medicine* a total of 520 times. With 520 as the numerator and 250 as the denominator (520/250), the impact factor would be a bit over 2. Impact factors for journals are reported annually in an SCI spin-off publication, the JCR (*Journal Citation Reports*). Other tallies from JCR are the ''Cited Half-Life'' and the ''Immediacy Factor.'' These numbers relate to how many years articles from a journal continue to be cited and how quickly articles are cited after publication. This gives you some quantifiable elements to use in your decisions for journal selections.

COST OF JOURNALS

The price of a journal certainly has to be a factor in your purchasing decision. Journals in the biomedical field are expensive. For the last few years, EBSCO, a serials jobber, has been doing studies of medical journal prices. "The total 1995 cost of the 2,547 *Index Medicus* titles with set annual subscription rates is $919,242.39. This represents a 51.4 percent increase over 1991 when there were 2,386 priced titles totaling just over $600,000. . . . the rise in average title price from $135.58 in 1986 to $360.91 in 1995" (Fortney and Basile 1995, 4). The study also provides groupings of journal titles within broad subject areas, and this demonstrates some strikingly high prices as well as great variations. For example, the average price in 1995 was $998.59 for the 55 biochemistry journals and $839.73 for the 26 neurosciences titles. Near the other end of the scale of prices, the 15 rehabilitation journals averaged $148.07, and the 37 nursing titles, $110.14. A subscription to *Brain Research* costs over $10,000, whereas the *Journal of Rehabilitation* is about $40 per year. A study was done on the price changes of the medical journals from the Brandon list. Also known as Brandon-Hill, this is a selected list of books and journals (it will be discussed in Chapter 4). This has a more restricted group of about 100 titles that would likely be found in even the smallest medical libraries. The average price in 1965, $13.90; in 1975, $29.71; in 1985, $70.46; and in 1995, $181.78 (Brandon and Hill 1995). This Brandon list has been published every other year in the April issue of the *Bulletin of the Medical Library Association*. The April 15 issue of *Library Journal* each year contains convenient price information on journals and discussions of factors in price increases, such as the value of the dollar compared to other currencies (Ketcham and Born 1995).

PUBLISHERS AND PRICES

The last ten years have witnessed a growing outcry by librarians over the very high prices charged for science journals. A feeling of being exploited, especially by foreign medical publishers, has led librarians to discuss cancellations, boycotts, and electronic revolutions. These conversations take place at meetings, in library periodicals, and now in electronic discussion groups and newsletters; for example, *The Newsletter on Serials Pricing Issues* is available over the Internet from the University of North Carolina (Tuttle). Serials librarians have developed a fourteen-point plan to address their problems with publishers and vendors (Quinn and Rogers 1992). Those points include the following issues: If libraries pursue large-scale cancellations, they will be relying more and more on satisfying their patrons' needs by outside sources. The oft-mentioned phrase "access over ownership" will be the reality. What does that mean for the future of our libraries? Since foreign for-profit publishers have taken a large part of the science journal market, can American research authors be encouraged to put pressure on those publishers who charge such high prices?

Librarians can also encourage authors to think in terms of the prices of the journals when they are submitting their research for publication. To librarians, the situation has seemed so unfair and unnecessary. After all, much of the research published in the journals is funded by the U.S. government. The journal editors are often scientists working at American universities. Why, then, do commercial publishers, especially foreign commercial publishers, often take over?

A broader look at medical journal publishing is called for. Pricing is important, but we need to know more. We know that the journals cost a lot of money and we have a vague sense of their importance to our patrons, but we must consider more. How are different types of journals used? What features are in different types of journals? (See Tony Stankus [1987, 1992] for more detailed information on the utility of specific journals, to understand their contributions and how they are used.) And who are the publishers of biomedical journals? Here is one way to categorize the different types of publishers, listed here with a representative publisher and journal:

1. Professional Societies—American College of Physicians (*Annals of Internal Medicine*)
2. University Presses—Cambridge University Press (*Journal of Physiology*)
3. Domestic For-Profit Presses—Lippincott (*Clinical Orthopaedics and Related Research*)
4. Foreign For-Profit Presses—Elsevier (*Biochimica et Biophysica Acta*)

Diverse organizations comprise medical publishing. How do they determine journal prices, about which we are so concerned? A for-profit commercial publisher may ask whatever price the market will bear; that is, publishers will keep raising prices as long as libraries continue to pay them. Publishers consider a variety of factors when establishing a pricing policy: (1) number of subscribers to the journal; (2) advertising revenue, which is based on the number of subscribers; and (3) number of pages. For the publishers, prices can be justified by economic forces. From the librarians' perspective, however, the situation is lamented: "The Least Amount for the Fewest Number at the Highest Prices." As the fields of specialization become narrower and narrower, the number of readers becomes fewer and fewer. Some of the most specialized journals have very high prices and small audiences. Note below, in particular, the basic research journal.

CATEGORIES OF BIOMEDICAL JOURNALS

1. General medical journals have very large subscriptions of 100,000 or so. They usually accept advertising, and their price may be under \$100. For example, *Annals of Internal Medicine* has a circulation of 95,000, comes out twice per month, is published by a professional society, has advertising, and costs \$92.

(Much of this data on the journals comes from *Ulrich's International Periodicals Directory, 1994–95.*)

2. Clinical care specialty journals have large subscriptions, focus on direct patient care, often accept advertising, and often cost a little bit more than the general medical journals. The *American Journal of Cardiology* has a circulation of 30,050, comes out 24 times per year, accepts advertising, and costs libraries $95.

3. Clinical research journals are more costly and have fewer subscriptions than the general medical journals and the clinical care specialty journals. For example, *Circulation Research* comes out monthly, costs $207, takes advertising, and has a circulation of 3,750.

4. The basic research journal category is the one that makes you take notice and calls you to action. These journals have a moderate to low number of subscribers, usually do not accept advertising, and may have very high prices. For example, *Biochimica et Biophysica Acta* (BBA) costs $7,322. It comes out in ten sections on different topics (e.g., molecular basis of disease). The total number of issues in a year is about 125. Although BBA is on the high side of the pricing continuum, many basic research journals cost $1,000 or $2,000 per year. Some may have only a few hundred subscribers. Since the journals do not get much revenue from advertisements, their publishers do rely on library subscriptions for revenue.

Another factor may be involved in publication of science articles. Page charges may be used to shift costs of publication to the authors of the article. Authors are not only not paid for their contributions to the literature but may be required to pay a set amount for each page their article takes up in the journal. Journals with page charges should be able to charge less for subscriptions. When commercial publishers are involved and the prices are high, there are usually no page charges. The preceding showed a few ways to group journals: by publisher type and by general role. We may also look at journals by article type or function, as shown in the next section.

JOURNALS BY ARTICLE TYPE OR FUNCTION

The thousands of journals may also be divided in the following ways. A representative title is given with each group type.

1. Original research, basic—*Cellular and Molecular Neurobiology*
2. Original research, clinical—*Circulation*
3. Patient care—*American Heart Journal*
4. Reviews of the current literature—*Annual Review of Biochemistry*
5. Symposia proceedings—*American Review of Respiratory Disease*
6. Descriptions of research methods—*Methods in Enzymology*
7. Overview articles of a subject (especially useful for students)—*Trends in Genetics*

8. Historical or philosophical aspects of the field—*Perspectives in Biology and Medicine*
9. Legal issues in the field—*Legal Aspects of Medical Care*
10. Educational issues in the field (e.g., for medical educators, for nursing educators)—*Academic Medicine*
11. Economic perspective—*Milbank Quarterly*
12. Interdisciplinary coverage—*Social Science and Medicine*
13. Fast publication of research results (letters-type journal)—*Biochemical and Biophysical Research Communications*
14. Professional or occupational issues (e.g., employment, licensure, or meetings announcements)—*American Journal of Nursing*
15. Current awareness and/or abstracts of the literature—*Current Contents: Clinical Medicine*

This list of journals by article type should not be construed to imply that all articles in a journal need to be of one type. Many journals set aside sections for particular purposes such as review articles and abstracts of meetings. In the library, we sometimes focus in on issues such as dual pricing, monopolistic practices, price gouging, and exchange rates of foreign currencies. It is important to be informed about these issues. However, we also need to understand the varieties and roles of different journals.

ACCESS: INTERLIBRARY LOAN AND DOCUMENT DELIVERY

Another factor in your decision to subscribe to a journal is its availability from other sources. With interlibrary loan, you have access to library collections across the country. For some immediate needs, you may be able to rely on libraries very close by. The union list showing journals held by the libraries in your consortium is a great help here. Use your interlibrary loan records as another tool to aid in the purchasing decision. You may be repeatedly requesting articles from the same journal. Libraries are required to keep records of interlibrary loan borrowing of photocopies, so this information will not be difficult to find. Under the current copyright guidelines, each year you may borrow up to five articles from a journal's current five years. It is easy to view this copyright regulation as a nuisance and an obstruction of the free interchange of information. Realistically, however, if you are borrowing a title often, it usually makes sense to subscribe to it. What do you do when you need ten or twenty articles per year from a very expensive journal? That number of articles exceeds what the copyright guidelines allow. On the other hand, you cannot justify spending over $7,000 on *Biochimica et Biophysica Acta* for a few dozen articles. This is the time to remember that the guidelines do not prohibit you from copying. The prohibition concerns excessive copying without compensation. Seemingly, this would be the occasion to note the dollar figures that appeared on the bottom of the first page of some journal articles several years ago. Many copyrighted journals now attach prices of $5.00 or $10.00 or more to an article. If you go beyond the limit of five, you could send in payment to either the publisher or a copyright clearance center. Now there are several document delivery organizations, such as UnCover or the Institute for Scientific Information (ISI), and they add in the copyright fee when they send you the article.

''Document delivery'' is a term applied to mechanisms of obtaining articles outside the library-to-library channels. Technology has a role to play here. Fax transmission is one means of document delivery. Computer scanning of text for transmission is another. The Medical Library Association meeting in May 1993 in Chicago presented a program entitled ''DocuShock: Options for Document Delivery in the '90s.'' It included explanations of Ariel (Research Libraries Group); Faxon Finder/Faxon Xpress (Faxon, the serials vendor); SAIL (National Library of Medicine); and UnCover (Knight-Ridder Information). For journal articles, geographic proximity should not be a barrier to good and speedy service. These are ventures and experiments in document delivery, and what happens here will be interesting. Is this providing a path to more widespread electronic publishing and purchases of journals article by article instead of by annual subscription? Note the analysis of records gathered from DOCLINE (discussed further in Chapter 7). This is the NLM system used by most health sciences libraries for interlibrary loan. The National Library of Medicine found that more than 2 million requests are made annually, and 97% of them are for journal articles. Important to plans concerning the future of article-by-article acquisition, this study found that 76% of the articles were requested just once (Lacroix 1994).

SUBSCRIPTION DECISIONS

You have evaluated your library's needs and have familiarized yourself with the issues of biomedical journals. It is time to decide on renewals and subscriptions for the coming year. What is to be done with *Brain Research*? The 1995 subscription was for over $10,100. But the dollar has not been strong, and there will be another price increase this year. What will the price be for 1996? $11,000? $12,000? Your subscription to *Brain Research* is actually a package deal. Along with *Brain Research* you receive *Brain Research Reviews*, *Developmental Brain Research*, *Molecular Brain Research*, *Discussions in Neuroscience*, and *Cognitive Brain Research*. You check the data in JCR, and these serials are among the most highly cited neuroscience journals. The field of neuroscience is very important at your institution. However, individual faculty and researchers volunteer the information that *Brain Research* is not really at the very top of neuroscience journals. In other words, it is not where they would typically go first to have their articles published. You check at the shelving stations. Volumes of *Brain Research* are there every day waiting to be reshelved.

This is true for both the current issues and the bound volumes of past years. *Brain Research* and its associated titles are thoroughly covered in the CD-ROM indexes your patrons use the most.

Where do you come out on this? *Brain Research* is outrageously expensive. People in the neuroscience department say it is OK to cancel. They have several journals they want the library to subscribe to and feel that a cancellation to *Brain Research* will free up a lot of money. If the average neuroscience journal costs about $1,000, perhaps ten other journals may be purchased. When someone needs an article from *Brain Research*, the library can buy it through document delivery at perhaps $10–$20 per article. You can buy a lot of articles for $10,000. But what about the demand? Students, faculty, and researchers are using *Brain Research* continuously throughout the day. Can we serve that level of demand with document delivery? You will need to arrive at a decision by weighing the benefits and the costs.

The medical school library at the Washington University in St. Louis did just that (Washington University 1993). They conducted a careful journal use study for the period July 1992 through June 1993 and found that *Brain Research* was not a bad deal. From its 1993 price of $9,484.33, it had 1,696 uses. This came to $5.59 per use. According to their studies, it would cost $26.00 (including the copyright fee) to obtain *Brain Research* through an article-by-article transaction. The $5.59 was not out of line with many other journals in the collection, such as *Life Sciences*, $6.56; *Neuroscience*, $6.29; and *Journal of Immunological Methods*, $5.99. Compare those to ones near the extremes of cost per use: *Carbohydrate Research*, $30.96; *Journal of Biological Chemistry*, $0.10.

Although these were data for one medical school library only, the numbers are interesting and may be instructive. You will need to base your calculations and decisions on the use in your library. Perhaps those ten other neuroscience journals you could subscribe to were *Brain Research* cancelled would be so heavily used in your library that their cumulative cost would be $2.00 per use. The opportunity cost, in the vocabulary of the economists, would be high for *Brain Research* because the cost of the journal crowds out the alternative, more effective use of funds.

BUDGETING

Determinations have been made on what journals need to be acquired for the collection to support your users. You have your list of 200 or 500 or 1,000 or 2,000 journal titles. The total dollar figure for the journal collection is large. Indeed, it will take the majority of the materials budget. That is reasonable, since the journals are your most important publications. However, as your journal payments go up and up, you may find that you run out of money for other things such as books. This is another issue to confront. The choices are limited. You must try to get more funds to support your journal habit or you will need to cut back on either book purchases or journal subscriptions. With increasing journal prices comes a real possibility that the book budget may completely disappear if no decisions are made to control the journals.

For a number of years, inflation has been greater here than for library materials in general, which has, in turn, been greater than the general average inflation for the country, the consumer price index. Remember, again, that you support the needs of your institution. If your institution is no longer involved in a particular subject, you probably cannot afford to keep subscribing to journals specific to that topic. You could very well feel that you have a nice run of a journal from volume 1 on, and it would be a shame to cancel it now. Unfortunately, this is not a satisfactory reason in the current climate of journals and economics.

AN ELECTRONIC SOLUTION?

The rapid publication of findings—with pictures and even sound, too—in an approved, established, accredited electronic medium may become a solution to a variety of problems and issues. The electronic format does not have to be a barrier to peer review. Quite to the contrary, it might facilitate that process. Some journals are now published simultaneously in paper and electronically, that is, on CD-ROM. A real issue to be addressed is the free-for-all phenomenon of much of the information available on the Internet. The most prestigious journal in medicine has come down firmly on this issue. While encouraging physicians to increase their competence in electronic communication, Kassirer and Angell (1995) will not endorse the posting of manuscripts to the Internet. Those manuscripts miss the rigorous peer review, they maintain. In addition, a full manuscript ''published'' on the Internet will not be considered for publication by the *New England Journal of Medicine*. Under the Ingelfinger Rule, it will have already been publicly disseminated. Note, too, that in 1996, the abstracts of some articles and the full text of others in the *New England Journal of Medicine* became available for free at the Web site, http://www.nejm.org. We will want to look at the promise of electronic journals and the Internet in Chapters 4 and 6. However, one practical problem we can confidently envision being solved by the electronic journal is this question from your physician or researcher: ''Where is the Green Journal?'' Experience may be the best resource for the answer to this question. However, here is a tip: Fenske and Fortney (1986) provide a clever list of ''green journals,'' ''gray books,'' ''red index,'' and the like.

One factor in deciding to subscribe to a journal is its coverage by the abstracting and indexing services. That directly affects information retrieval and the demand for the articles. Chapters 2 and 3 examine this.

2

Indexing, *Index Medicus*, and Other Traditional Abstracting and Indexing Services

THE NEED FOR INDEXING AND INDEXES

Chapter 1 included the biomedical journal in its role in communicating research findings to other researchers and to the providers of health care. With thousands of journals and hundreds of thousands of journal articles produced each year, individual physicians may, for example, find it very difficult to obtain exactly the information they need to treat each patient. The problem of keeping up to date is not new, of course. Even in this era of computerized databases, health practitioners do not always get the information they need. Why is that? What is the information-seeking behavior of physicians? Of most people? If they have a question, they may check their own collections of books and journals. If that proves unsatisfactory, they may ask colleagues. Finally, they may approach the literature. The medical literature is underused (Huth 1989). This is particularly unfortunate because often the literature contains useful answers. What must we as librarians do to solve the problem? We have to make it easier to find the information.

Overall, this is rather disappointing news because finding information has already been made much easier. Many people, scientists and physicians among them, have large databases of information at their fingertips. The databases are available via telephone lines or via dedicated lines or found on locally mounted computers or on nearby optical storage devices or accessed through the Internet. The information is as close as the computers on their desks. Is this not easy enough? Availability of information may not be the relevant issue. The riches of information available actually help keep the individual physician relatively information poor. The answer we in the library have traditionally offered to make this wealth of information manageable is indexing. The primary tools we have to search the biomedical literature are the abstracting and indexing services. Thus a thorough understanding of the indexing process and the indexes is a must for the medical librarian. Having accepted that, perhaps we need to take a longer-term view. Maybe we will not always have to learn indexing principles and practices. The combination of full-text databases with statistical analyses of texts may enable us to obtain the information we want just by using about any type of English-language query. This is in fact happening. However, perhaps it is not happening quickly enough, and so a close look at current practice is in order. Although we use paper indexes less and less, the principles of organization and storage of information applied to paper indexes are used with computer searching as well. In other words, you still need to understand the indexing process. This chapter concentrates on the print products, but some mention of computer counterparts is necessary here, too. (Chapter 3 more fully examines the computerized indexes.)

INDEX MEDICUS AND MESH

Index Medicus is the most important print tool for accessing the medical literature. The computerized counterpart of IM is MEDLINE. MEDLINE's coverage is somewhat larger in that it includes more nursing and dental journals than IM. *Index Medicus* covers over 3,000 biomedical periodicals. Although that number sounds large and is large, many health sciences journals are not included in it. In addition, many journals in related fields such as chemistry, physics, and psychology that have information that bears on the science of biology and the practice of medicine are not in IM. Around 30,000 articles are included in each of the monthly issues of IM. At the end of the year, the *Cumulated Index Medicus* is compiled. *Index Medicus* contains an author index and a subject index. The vocabulary for the subject index comes from the thesaurus, *Medical Subject Headings* (MeSH). In addition, there are MeSH publications designed for searching MEDLINE: (1) *Medical Subject Headings—Annotated Alphabetic List*, (2) *Medical Subject Headings—Tree Structures,* and (3) *Permuted Medical Subject Headings.* MeSH has over 17,000 main headings to describe the contents of the journal articles. Over 75 subheadings are available to specify aspects of the main MeSH entries. Therefore, for any month or year, a physician, researcher, nurse, librarian, student, or anyone else could go to the subject index to look for articles on the specific topic desired.

Figure 2.1 has an entry from the subject index of the July 1992 issue of IM. The entries are arranged in alphabetical order by MeSH. If the index user were looking in the *S*'s for ''slipped disk,'' he would be guided to the heading ''INTERVERTEBRAL DISK DISPLACEMENT.''

Figure 2.1
Index Medicus

Disc degeneration and angular movement of the lumbar spine: comparative study using plain and flexion-extension radiography and discography. Soini J, et al. **J Spinal Disord** 1991 Jun;4(2):183-7
Measurement variations in scoliotic angle, vertebral rotation, vertebral body height, and intervertebral disc space height. Ylikoski M, et al. **J Spinal Disord** 1990 Dec;3(4):387-91
Cervical disc calcification in children. A long-term review. Wong CC, et al. **Spine** 1992 Feb;17(2):139-44

SURGERY

Discitis after lumbar disc surgery. Features of "aseptic" and "septic" forms. Fouquet B, et al. **Spine** 1992 Mar; 17(3):356-8
[Cervical disk defects. Results of surgical treatment of cervical vertebral radiculopathy] Wiberg J. **Tidsskr Nor Laegeforen** 1992 Mar 10;112(7):876-80 (Eng. Abstr.) **(Nor)**

INTERVERTEBRAL DISK DISPLACEMENT

see related
SCIATICA
Intradural disc herniations in the cervical, thoracic, and lumbar spine: report of three cases and review of the literature. Epstein NE, et al. **J Spinal Disord** 1990 Dec; 3(4):396-403 (23 ref.)

COMPLICATIONS

Thoracic disk herniation and recurrent dislocation of total hip prosthesis. Bunning RD, et al. **South Med J** 1992 Apr; 85(4):416-8
[A case report of cervical disc hernia presenting fecal incontinence evoked by walking, spinal intermittent rectal dysfunction] Mizuno M, et al. **No Shinkei Geka** 1992 Apr; 20(4):445-9 (Eng. Abstr.) **(Jpn)**
[Epidural injections of steroids in the treatment of patients with chronic sciatica in discopathy] Popiołek A, et al. **Neurol Neurochir Pol** 1991 Sep-Oct;25(5):640-6 (Eng. Abstr.) **(Pol)**

DIAGNOSIS

Clinical MR imaging of degenerative spinal disease: pulse sequences, gradient-echo techniques, and contrast agents. Ross JS, et al. **J Magn Reson Imaging** 1991 Jan-Feb; 1(1):29-37 (42 ref.)
Use of magnetic resonance imaging in the decision-making process for lumbar intervertebral disc syndrome. Robinson GK. **J Manipulative Physiol Ther** 1992 Feb;15(2):129-32
MRI classification of lumbar herniated intervertebral disc. Kim KY, et al. **Orthopedics** 1992 Apr;15(4):493-7

ECONOMICS

Cost-effectiveness analysis of extended conservative therapy versus surgical intervention in the management of herniated lumbar intervertebral disc. Shvartzman L, et al. **Spine** 1992 Feb;17(2):176-82

ETIOLOGY

The role and incidence of facet tropism in lumbar spine degenerative disc disease. Murtagh FR, et al. **J Spinal Disord** 1991 Mar;4(1):86-9
A herniated cervical disc resulting from discography: an unusual complication. Smith MD, et al. **J Spinal Disord** 1990 Dec;3(4):392-4; discussion 395

PHYSIOPATHOLOGY

Influence of disc degeneration on mechanism of thoracolumbar burst fractures. Shirado O, et al. **Spine** 1992 Mar;17(3):286-92

SURGERY

Anterior microsurgical approach for degenerative cervical disc disease. Klaiber RD, et al. **Acta Neurochir (Wien)** 1992; 114(1-2):36-42
Herniated lumbar disc in patients over the age of fifty. An HS, et al. **J Spinal Disord** 1990 Jun;3(2):143-6
The treatment of lumbar disc herniation: simple fragment excision versus disc space curettage. Balderston RA, et al. **J Spinal Disord** 1991 Mar;4(1):22-5
Clinical factors predicting outcome after surgery for herniated lumbar disc: an epidemiological multivariate analysis. Barrios C, et al. **J Spinal Disord** 1990 Sep; 3(3):205-9
Redecompression and fusion in failed back syndrome patients. Biondi J, et al. **J Spinal Disord** 1990 Dec;3(4):362-9
Benefits of epidural methylprednisolone in a unilateral lumbar discectomy: a matched controlled study. Davis R, et al. **J Spinal Disord** 1990 Dec;3(4):299-306; discussion 307 (27 ref.)
Surgically confirmed cauda equina and nerve root injury following percutaneous discectomy at an outside institution: a case report. Epstein NE. **J Spinal Disord** 1990 Dec;3(4):380-2; discussion 383 (11 ref.)
Acute complications in patients with surgical treatment of lumbar herniated disc. Kardaun JW, et al. **J Spinal Disord** 1990 Mar;3(1):30-8 (38 ref.)
Ceramic interspinous block (CISB) assisted anterior interbody fusion. Tsuji H, et al. **J Spinal Disord** 1990 Mar; 3(1):77-86
Results of lumbosacral fusion for degenerative disc disease with and without instrumentation. Two- to five-year follow-up. Grubb SA, et al. **Spine** 1992 Mar;17(3):349-55
Far lateral lumbar disc herniation treated with an anterolateral retroperitoneal approach. Report of two cases. Strum PF, et al. **Spine** 1992 Mar;17(3):363-5
[Good results in reoperation of recurrent radicular syndrome following surgery for herniated nucleus pulposus] van Burken MM, et al. **Ned Tijdschr Geneeskd** 1992 Apr 4; 136(14):692-5 (Eng. Abstr.) **(Dut)**
[Prevention of thromboembolism complications with low molecular weight heparin in microneurosurgical lumbar intervertebral disk operations] Prestar FJ. **Neurochirurgia (Stuttg)** 1992 Jan;35(1):1-4 (Eng. Abstr.) **(Ger)**
[Regression of motor symptoms after intervertebral disk displacement-induced spinal nerve root lesion. Clinical study] Mohsenipour I, et al. **Wien Klin Wochenschr** 1992; 104(3):61-6 (Eng. Abstr.) **(Ger)**
[Surgical treatment of lumbar disk prolapse. A 20-year material] Fiane AE, et al. **Tidsskr Nor Laegeforen** 1992 Jan 30;112(3):325-7 (Eng. Abstr.) **(Nor)**
[Posterior lumbar fusion using spongious-metal pins in lumbar instability and spondylolisthesis] Ugrinovski J, et al. **Reumatizam** 1991;38(5-6):19-22 (Eng. Abstr.) **(Scr)**

INTERVIEW, PSYCHOLOGICAL

[The five-minute interview. A brief method for assessing expressed emotion status] Stark FM, et al. **Nervenarzt** 1992 Jan;63(1):42-5 (Eng. Abstr.) **(Ger)**
[Symptom portrayal and initial therapeutic relationship of female and male patients in the initial psychoanalytic interview] Grande T, et al. **Z Psychosom Med Psychoanal** 1992;38(1):31-48 (Eng. Abstr.) **(Ger)**
[Compliance in epilepsy. II. Practical aspects] Alonso NB, et al. **Arq Neuropsiquiatr** 1991 Jun;49(2):150-4 (Eng. Abstr.) **(Por)**

INTERVIEWER EFFECT see **EFFECT MODIFIERS (EPIDEMIOLOGY)**

INTERVIEWS

Questionnaire versus clinical interview in the diagnosis of headache [letter] Lipton RB, et al. **Headache** 1992 Jan; 32(1):55-6
Contaminant identification: the importance of thorough interviewing techniques. Mrvos R, et al. **Vet Hum Toxicol** 1991 Dec;33(6):611-2

METHODS

Analysis of sexual behaviour in France (ACSF). A comparison between two modes of investigation: telephone survey and face-to-face survey. ASCF principal investigators and their associates [see comments] **AIDS** 1992 Mar;6(3):315-23. Comment in: AIDS 1992 Mar;6(3):329-23.
Understanding sexual behaviour [editorial; comment] McQueen D. **AIDS** 1992 Mar;6(3):329-30. Comment on: AIDS 1992 Mar;6(3):315-23.
The use of ethnographic interviewing to inform questionnaire construction. Bauman LJ, et al. **Health Educ Q** 1992 Spring; 19(1):9-23

INTESTINAL ABSORPTION

see related
MALABSORPTION SYNDROMES
Nonlinearities in amoxycillin pharmacokinetics. II. Absorption studies in the rat. Torres-Molina F, et al. **Biopharm Drug Dispos** 1992 Jan;13(1):39-53
The diagnostic value of the D-xylose absorption test in horses with unexplained chronic weight loss. Brown CM. **Br Vet J** 1992 Jan-Feb;148(1):41-4
Influence of food on the oral absorption and bioavailability of moricizine. Pieniaszek HJ Jr, et al. **J Clin Pharmacol** 1991 Sep;31(9):792-5
Comparison of absorption of erythorbic acid and ascorbic acid in guinea pig small intestine. Suzuki E, et al. **J Nutr Sci Vitaminol (Tokyo)** 1991 Oct;37(5):453-9
Normalization of vitamin B12 absorption after ileal resection in children. Ooi BC, et al. **J Paediatr Child Health** 1992 Apr;28(2):168-71
Gastrointestinal citrate absorption in nephrolithiasis. Fegan J, et al. **J Urol** 1992 May;147(5):1212-4
Gastrointestinal function in obesity: motility, secretion, and absorption following a liquid test meal. Wisén O, et al. **Metabolism** 1992 Apr;41(4):390-5
Absorption of oligo-L-[35S]methionine after feeding of a low casein or a low soybean protein isolate diet in rats. Hara H, et al. **Proc Soc Exp Biol Med** 1992 May;200(1):30-5
The [14C]-triolein breath test is not valid as a test of fat absorption. Pedersen NT, et al. **Scand J Clin Lab Invest** 1991 Dec;51(8):699-703
Net absorption of water, electrolytes, glucose, and folate from the in vivo, neurally isolated canine jejunum. Hakim NS, et al. **Surgery** 1992 Apr;111(4):394-401
The piglet as a model animal for studying aspects of digestion and absorption in milk-fed human infants. Moughan PJ, et al. **World Rev Nutr Diet** 1992;67:40-113 (317 ref.)

DRUG EFFECTS

Rapid stimulation of intestinal D-glucose transport in teleosts by 17 alpha-methyltestosterone. Hazzard CE, et al. **Am J Physiol** 1992 Mar;262(3 Pt 2):R412-8
Investigation of the possible influence of the absorption of vinpocetine with concomitant application of magnesium-aluminium-hydroxide gel. Lohmann A, et al. **Arzneimittelforschung** 1991 Nov;41(11):1164-7
Intestinal absorption of copper: influence of carbohydrates. Wapnir RA, et al. **Biochem Med Metab Biol** 1992 Feb; 47(1):47-53
Enhancement effect of lauric acid on the rectal absorption of propranolol from suppository in rats. Ogiso T, et al. **Chem Pharm Bull (Tokyo)** 1991 Oct;39(10):2657-61
Intestinal follow-through examinations with iohexol and iopentol. Permeability alterations and efficacy in patients with small bowel obstruction. Laerum F, et al. **Invest Radiol** 1991 Nov;26 Suppl 1:S177-81; discussion S185
Effect of 24,25-dihydroxycholecalciferol on intestinal absorption of calcium and phosphate and on parathyroid hormone secretion in chronic renal failure. Varghese Z, et al. **Nephron** 1992;60(3):286-91
Enhanced bioavailability of cefoxitin using palmitoyl L-carnitine. I. Enhancer activity in different intestinal regions. Sutton SC, et al. **Pharm Res** 1992 Feb;9(2):191-4
[Study of combined effects of mixtures of pesticides from various chemical groups on calcium absorption in the rat intestine. I. Dichlorvos and thiram] Witkowska D, et al. **Rocz Panstw Zakl Hig** 1991;42(2):171-7 (Eng. Abstr.) **(Pol)**
[The effect of regulatory peptides on water absorption in the large intestine of the frog] Barashkova GM, et al. **Fiziol Zh** 1992 Jan-Feb;38(1):57-63 (Eng. Abstr.) **(Rus)**

PHYSIOLOGY

Rat intestinal amino acid balances after the administration of an oral protein load. Fernández-López JA, et al. **Biochem Int** 1992 Feb;26(2):297-308
Relevance of physiology of nutrient absorption to formulation of enteral diets. Silk DB, et al. **Nutrition** 1992 Jan-Feb;8(1):1-12 (132 ref.)
The role of calcium metabolism abnormalities in the development of ossification of the posterior longitudinal ligament of the cervical spine. Seichi A, et al. **Spine** 1992 Mar;17(3 Suppl):S30-2
[Colon helps short bowel syndrome] Michel P. **Gastroenterol Clin Biol** 1992;16(2):195-6 **(Fre)**

INTESTINAL AMEBIASIS see **DYSENTERY, AMEBIC**

INTESTINAL ATRESIA

COMPLICATIONS

Duodenal atresia presenting as hematemesis in a premature infant with Down syndrome. Case report and review of the literature. Chhabra R, et al. **J Perinatol** 1992 Mar; 12(1):25-7 (12 ref.)

INTESTINAL DISEASES

CHEMICALLY INDUCED

Senna and pseudomelanosis coli. **Pharmacology** 1992;44 Suppl 1:33-5

COMPLICATIONS

Autoimmune enteropathy, anti-tubular basement membrane antibodies, and glomerulonephritis [letter] Levy M. **J Pediatr** 1992 Apr;120(4 Pt 1):659

DIAGNOSIS

Small bowel endoscopy. Waye JD. **Endoscopy** 1992 Jan-Feb; 24(1-2):68-72 (19 ref.)
[Hepatic and intestinal sequelae of inflammatory vascular processes] Poralla T. **Verh Dtsch Ges Inn Med** 1991; 97:525-9 (16 ref.) **(Ger)**
[Diagnosis of small intestinal diseases] Parfenov AI, et al. **Klin Med (Mosk)** 1991 Nov;69(11):103-7 (30 ref.) **(Rus)**
[Ways to improve the diagnosis and treatment of patients with acute intestinal infections at the prehospital stage] Mashilov VP, et al. **Ter Arkh** 1991;63(11):10-1 (Eng. Abstr.) **(Rus)**

ETIOLOGY

Systemic elastolytic granulomatosis with cutaneous, ocular, lymph nodal, and intestinal involvement. Spectrum of annular elastolytic giant cell granuloma and sarcoidosis. Kurose N, et al. **J Am Acad Dermatol** 1992 Feb;26(2 Pt 2):359-63
[A prospective study of chronic radiation lesions of the small intestine after radiotherapy of gynecologic cancer] Moschoutis P, et al. **Ann Gastroenterol Hepatol (Paris)** 1992 Jan-Feb;28(1):1-6 (Eng. Abstr.) **(Fre)**

slipped disk see intervertebral disk displacement

Under the headings are subheadings in smaller type. Entries for journal articles include the title, first author, journal abbreviation, date, volume, issue, and page range. The titles with brackets around them are for articles not written in English. Some of the foreign-language articles have the note ''Eng. Abstr.'' This alerts the reader that although the article is not in English, there is an English language abstract included with the article. Some entries have a note about the number of other publications to which that journal article refers (e.g., ''177 ref.''). This signals a review-type article that often surveys the current literature written on that subject. Another publication helpful in the use of IM is the *List of Journals Indexed in Index Medicus*. This publication includes a list of the abbreviations used for the journals with the full spellings of the title. Here is a sample entry from the author index of the July 1992 IM.

Balderston RA, Gilyard GG, Jones AA, Wiesel SW, Spengler DM, Bigos SJ, Rothman RH. The treatment of lumbar disc herniation: simple fragment excision versus disc space curettage. *J Spine Disord* 1991 Mar;4(1):22–5.

Authors' names are given last name first. Initials of first and middle names are included. Only the initials are used in the IM citation. The initials are taken from the names on the journal article itself. Therefore, if an author sometimes includes a middle name or initial on his or her papers and sometimes does not, slightly different forms of his or her name are in the index. The authority control familiar to librarians for personal names in cataloging of books for card or online catalogs is not used in most periodical indexes. This may not pose a great problem in the print index because the array of choices is obvious at a glance. However, with computer searching you may miss citations if you do not keep in mind this indexing practice. Up to ten authors of an article are included, with two through ten having a ''see reference'' back to the first author. (In 1996, the maximum number of authors increased to include up to 25.) In the *G*'s, there is this entry:

Gilyard GG see Balderston RA

Then come the title of the journal article, journal abbreviation, date, volume, issue, and pages. Foreign-language articles are not in brackets here but do have a three-letter designation (e.g., Ger).

INDEXING AND SUBJECT ACCESS

Why is it important for librarians to understand the indexing process? An authorized language can bring together information on a topic regardless of how the author described a condition: slipped disk and herniated disk and intervertebral disk displacement; myopia and nearsightedness; kidney stones and renal calculi; diabetes and diabetic retinopathy; rodents and rats; cancer and neoplasms; drug therapy and chemotherapy; etiology and cause. There is no authority that tells researchers or health practitioners what words they must use to describe the biomedical conditions they are writing about in their journal articles. Richness of language enhances conversation and literature. However, it also creates obstacles to satisfactory information retrieval. True, a language of a discipline is specialized; for example, cardiologists are less likely to use the lay term "heart attack." Still, practitioners of the discipline do not always use the same terms, and it is unlikely that individuals will accept a uniform mode of expression in their writing. We, as information retrieval specialists, must provide a dependable and easy way to eliminate these problems to help people get what they need.

In order to search the literature efficiently, we need to familiarize ourselves with the indexing vocabulary and the rules indexers use when assigning subject headings. Because librarians, physicians, and other health practitioners do depend on IM and MEDLINE to access the biomedical literature, we need to look at MeSH carefully. Our examples (myopia and nearsightedness) may give the impression that the control of synonyms would solve the problem. Actually, several difficulties must be addressed, including the need to control synonyms, in order to create an effective searching vocabulary. The rules used by indexers at the National Library of Medicine (NLM) are designed to help solve those problems. Parenthetically, it should be noted that these rules of indexing will not stay the same forever. Better ways to retrieve information will be developed, just as we assume there will be improved treatments for the patients' diseases. In other words, what follows does not represent something that you cannot and will not improve upon.

CHOICE OF TERMS IN MESH

Let's say that a journal article discusses diseases of the heart. Disregard momentarily that this is a large topic that is too general for most papers. (Also note, for this chapter and the next, MeSH headings appear in all capitals.) What MeSH term should be used? For this topic, a searcher for information may look at: HEART, HEART DISEASES, and CARDIOLOGY. Terms like CARDIOVASCULAR DISEASES may also come to mind. All are MeSH entries. HEART is the anatomical term. HEART DISEASES is the disease term. CARDIOLOGY is the medical specialty entry. Indexers and searchers have been warned against using the medical specialty. The disease term is preferable. The medical specialty entry has been reserved for issues relating to the practice of that area of medicine (e.g., training needed to become a cardiologist, malpractice concerns of cardiologists). The term CARDIOLOGY is not used for diagnosis and treatment of cardiovascular problems. This is one indexing guideline. How are terms selected for the vocabulary? In each issue of IM, the introduction gives the following tips for finding the appropriate subject terms:

Because it is impossible to group together all terms directly or indirectly related to a particular concept, the following should be considered when searching this bibliography:

1. Direct form of a term (LUNG ABSCESS)
2. Inverted form of a term (ANEMIA, HEMOLYTIC)
3. Noun form (LIVER; KIDNEY; BRAIN)
4. Adjective form (HEPATIC VEINS, CEREBRAL REVASCULARIZATION)
5. Consider also references printed under several headings
6. Function words which imply the concept in mind (THINKING for BRAIN, DIGESTION for DIGESTIVE SYSTEM)
7. Terms for techniques which imply the concept in mind (ELECTROCARDIOGRAPHY for HEART)
8. Synonyms or near-synonyms (JOHNE'S DISEASE see PARATUBERCULOSIS)
9. Broader or narrower terms

(National Library of Medicine 1995e: viii–ix)

From this it seems clear that you might not be able to guess the MeSH heading by relying on your subject expertise or even by knowing the terms often used in the journal literature. You will need to look up the possibilities in MeSH.

THE INDEXING PROCESS, SPECIFICITY, AND TREES

The indexer at NLM first looks at the title to grasp the author's main points. Next, a reading of the introductory material should further convey what the author hopes to demonstrate. Scanning the methods, results, and conclusions sections will reveal the substantive points of the article. Because many abstracts included by the author are not written informatively and may not accurately represent the articles of which they are a part, indexers read the abstract last only to double check any points they may have missed. In journal article indexing, the entire article is not read. The indexer decides which concepts are covered in the journal article, and the MeSH headings are used to select which headings should be assigned to describe those ideas.

The first rule in selecting the headings is specificity. Each term chosen is as specific as is warranted by the article. Let us say that an article discusses hepatitis. Hepatitis is a liver disease. HEPATITIS and LIVER DISEASES are both MeSH headings. The indexer will assign HEPATITIS to the article and not also LIVER DISEASES. If a library patron opened IM to the *L*'s to look for hepatitis under the heading LIVER DISEASES, would it be apparent that he or she was in the wrong place? Probably not. Some general articles on liver diseases do mention hepatitis. However, the bulk of hepatitis articles will not be found there. Would it be any more apparent from a computer terminal? A term is entered.

Citations are printed out. How would they know that there are many other relevant articles in the database?

At this point, let's look at MeSH. The MeSH that comes with the print IM is referred to as the Black and White MeSH (the colors of the cover—we are no different than the physicians with their ''Green Journal''). Terms are added and deleted each year, but for our purposes it should be sufficient to pick up any issue of the last few years. Although passages are displayed here, it may be useful to have the publications themselves at hand as you read through this. The terms are in alphabetical order and we will go to the *L*'s.

LIVER DISEASES
C6.552+

That alphanumeric designation ''C6.552+'' is the *Tree Number*. You then leave the alphabetic section and go to the *Tree Structures*. The *Tree Structures* arrange the MeSH headings in hierarchical groupings so that you can determine the general (broader) and specific (narrower) headings. The terms can be found by using that alphanumeric designation. Category C is ''Diseases.'' C6 is for Diseases-Digestive. At C6.552 there is LIVER DISEASES. Indented under LIVER DISEASES at C6.552.380 is HEPATITIS.

C6—Diseases-Digestive

LIVER DISEASES	C6.552
ACUTE YELLOW ATROPHY	C6.552.45
CHOLESTASIS, INTRAHEPATIC	C6.552.150
ALAGILLE SYNDROME	C6.552.150.125
LIVER CIRRHOSIS, BILIARY	C6.552.150.250
FATTY LIVER	C6.552.241
FATTY LIVER, ALCOHOLIC	C6.552.241.390
REYE'S SYNDROME	C6.552.241.649
HEPATIC VEIN THROMBOSIS	C6.552.347
HEPATIC VENO-OCCLUSIVE DISEASE	C6.552.360
HEPATITIS	C6.552.380
HEPATITIS, ALCOHOLIC	C6.552.380.290
HEPATITIS, ANIMAL	C6.552.380.315
HEPATITIS, VIRAL, ANIMAL	C6.552.380.315.430
HEPATITIS, INFECTIOUS CANINE	C6.552.380.315.430.440
RIFT VALLEY FEVER	C6.552.380.315.430.812
HEPATITIS, TOXIC	C6.552.380.615
HEPATITIS, VIRAL, HUMAN	C6.552.380.705

DELTA INFECTION	C6.552.380.705.270
HEPATITIS A	C6.552.380.705.422
HEPATITIS B	C6.552.380.705.437
HEPATITIS C	C6.552.380.705.440
HEPATITIS, CHRONIC ACTIVE	C6.552.380.705.460
HEPATITIS E	C6.552.380.705.470
HEPATOLENTICULAR DEGENERATION	C6.552.413
HEPATOMEGALY	C6.552.446
etc.	

Looking over the list of headings, you may find an even more specific and appropriate entry (e.g., DELTA INFECTION; HEPATITIS A). Taking a step back from the specific, here is a list of the general categories of the trees—how the MeSH terms are arranged.

A	ANATOMY
B	ORGANISMS
C	DISEASES
D	CHEMICALS AND DRUGS
E	ANALYTICAL, DIAGNOSTIC, AND THERAPEUTIC TECHNIQUES AND EQUIPMENT
F	PSYCHIATRY AND PSYCHOLOGY
G	BIOLOGICAL SCIENCES
H	PHYSICAL SCIENCES
I	ANTHROPOLOGY, EDUCATION, SOCIOLOGY, AND SOCIAL PHENOMENA
J	TECHNOLOGY, INDUSTRY, AGRICULTURE
K	HUMANITIES
L	INFORMATION SCIENCE
M	NAMED GROUPS
N	HEALTH CARE
Z	GEOGRAPHICALS

Classifying a disease or a chemical or a procedure or the other types of entries to just one category or tree is very difficult. Therefore, many headings are put in multiple locations in the *Tree Structures*. For example, the heading HEPATITIS, ALCOHOLIC is located not only where we saw it above but also at C6.552.645, where it is under LIVER DISEASES, ALCOHOLIC. Also, it is in category C21—Injury, Occupational Diseases, Poisoning. The *Tree Structures* include headings that are used for the indexing of articles. Back in the alphabetical listing we saw the ''see'' references (e.g., Slipped Disk see Intervertebral

Disk Displacement). However, not all the headings you might try to look up have been created and placed in alphabetical order. There is not a ''see'' reference for everything. It may therefore be useful to check one of the tools that usually goes with MEDLINE, *Permuted Medical Subject Headings*, which gives a listing for every word that appears in MeSH. Included, too, are words from ''see'' references, those entries that are used as guides to the preferred term. Here is the entry at ''Disk.''

Disk

Chemolysis, Intervertebral Disk see Intervertebral Disk Chemolysis

Choked Disk see Papilledema

Compact Disk Read-Only Memory see CD-ROM

Disk, Herniated see Intervertebral Disk Displacement

Disk, Intervertebral see Intervertebral Disk

Drusen, Optic Disk see Optic Disk Drusen

Intervertebral Disk

Intervertebral Disk Chemolysis

Intervertebral Disk Displacement

Nucleolysis, Intervertebral Disk see Intervertebral Disk Chemolysis

Optic Disk

Optic Disk Drusen

Prolapsed Disk see Intervertebral Disk Displacement

Slipped Disk see Intervertebral Disk Displacement

CHOICE OF HEADINGS: PRECOORDINATED HEADING AND MAIN HEADING WITH SUBHEADING

Take the case of an indexer examining an article covering liver diseases caused by parasites. There is the MeSH term LIVER and another one DISEASE and another one PARASITES. The indexer is not going to assign those terms to this article. When you look in IM under DISEASE, you will not find this article. There happens to be a precoordinated term, LIVER DISEASES, PARASITIC, and that is where this journal article belongs. While you are at it, you might as well check the trees to see if even more specific headings would be relevant.

LIVER DISEASES, PARASITIC	C6.552.664
ECHINOCOCCOSIS, HEPATIC	C6.552.664.272
FASCIOLIASIS	C6.552.664.424
LIVER ABSCESS, AMEBIC	C6.552.664.642

If no precoordinated heading is available to describe a topic, the indexer must check to see if a Main Heading–Subheading combination covers what you are interested in. For example, if the journal article discusses a cause of herniated disks, the indexer will assign the main heading INTERVERTEBRAL DISK DISPLACEMENT and put the subheading ''etiology'' with it. Look again at Figure 2.1. INTERVERTEBRAL DISK DISPLACEMENT is divided up by several subheadings, with ''etiology'' being one of them. If you look in MeSH or in other passages in IM, you will see that several of the subheadings also have the same word or phrase as a main MeSH heading (e.g., BLOOD, CYTOLOGY, DRUG THERAPY). The main heading DRUG THERAPY will not be used for an article like ''Drug Therapy of Slipped Disks.'' The subheading ''drug therapy'' would be used. The main heading DRUG THERAPY would be assigned to more general discussions of drug therapy. An example from the September 1992 issue of IM is found under the main heading DRUG THERAPY:

The effect of physician education on knowledge of drug therapeutics and costs. Sumpton JE, et al. Ann Pharmacother 1992 May;26(5):692–7.

MULTIPLICITY AND POSTCOORDINATION

Only at this point will an indexer assign separate main headings to describe the ideas of the article. If one article happens to discuss hepatitis and also herniated disks, the two separate headings HEPATITIS and INTERVERTEBRAL DISK DISPLACEMENT will be assigned. There is no precoordinated heading that would cover it—no term HEPATITIS AND INTERVERTEBRAL DISK DISPLACEMENT. There is no HEPATITIS–''intervertebral disk displacement'' as a heading-subheading combination either. Searching the print IM for an article covering both ideas, the patron would need to look under either HEPATITIS or INTERVERTEBRAL DISK DISPLACEMENT and scan the titles for the presence of the other idea.

Postcoordination refers to combining of terms by the searcher after the indexing is done. To do postcoordination manually is not very efficient and is also tedious. Postcoordination usually implies the use of the computer. *Index Medicus*'s computer counterpart, MEDLINE, would be a good choice here. The indexing vocabulary (MeSH) combined with the manipulation of headings by computer makes for a powerful searching system. The object of all this indexing is the journal article, and these articles in science and medicine are not very long—they are commonly five to ten pages. The number of MeSH headings assigned to one article is usually from ten to fifteen. Compare that to the one-to-four subject terms that are typically assigned to books of hundreds of pages when they are cataloged. A different strategy is involved in the cataloging of books. Each subject heading assigned is supposed to be descriptive of the whole book or, at least, a good part of it. That is not the case for journal articles. Using several headings for a relatively small work enables the indexer to describe the work in more depth. In addition, it serves the feature referred to as multiplicity, which is described this way in the *MEDLARS Indexing Manual*: ''Since MEDLARS is used by many types of research worker and clinician, the indexer will provide for each article as many subject headings as he deems necessary to index the article adequately from *all* its aspects. This is called multiple-indexing'' (Charen 1983, sect. 4, p. 4). By combining various terms when searching for information by computer, patrons or librarians can tailor the search to their detailed specifications. They will not find an article under all of those ten or so MeSH headings in the print IM. Note also that the indexers at NLM do not provide a separate group of terms for the print index and another group for the computer retrieval. The indexing for both is done simultaneously (Sewell 1964). The solution is *Index Medicus* and Non *Index Medicus*.

IM (*INDEX MEDICUS*), NIM (NON *INDEX MEDICUS*), AND CHECK TAGS

Only two, three, or four terms per article are coded by the indexer as ''IM.'' This means the article will appear under that subject heading in the paper subject index of IM. These headings reflect the main points of the articles listed. ''NIM'' is Non *Index Medicus*. Articles assigned a term at the NIM level do not appear under that subject heading in the paper IM. With so many headings assigned for computerized retrieval, the searcher can reach more deeply into an article, since ideas covered beyond the main points are also retrievable. The reason that the article is not placed under all the MeSH headings in the print IM is economic: Doing so would greatly enlarge the volumes and make them more expensive to produce. (Later in this chapter, we will consider some of the tribulations of producing the print IM.) The production of the paper index remains relatively expensive. In addition, the monthly subject index contains in the neighborhood of 1,500 pages. Recall from Chapter 1 the discussion of IM's size and David Durack's ''The Weight of Medical Knowledge.'' In that case, the weight was the weighing of the *Index Medicus* volumes on a scale.

Some concepts are very common and should therefore be assigned to a great percentage of articles in the database. For example, there are the age group headings. If the article discusses a disease in children who are four years old, the indexer must assign the term CHILD, PRESCHOOL. That designation covers children from two to six. If the article includes an experiment using rats, the indexer must assign the term ANIMAL as well as the regular term RATS. These types of general ideas are called ''check tags.'' On the indexing work form that had been used at NLM, the indexer did not need to find the appropriate terms for those general concepts in MeSH and then write them down. They were already on the indexing form and just needed to be ''checked.'' These days the form has been converted to the computer. Words that are used as check tags are almost always NIM and do not appear in the paper IM.

A JOURNAL ARTICLE AND ITS INDEXING

Consider the information about one of the articles listed in Figure 2.1:

Thoracic disk herniation and recurrent dislocation of total hip prosthesis. Bunning RD, et al. South Med J 1992 Apr;85(4):416–8.

These are the IM entries where you will find this article listed:

*HIP DISLOCATION at the subheading, etiology
*HIP PROSTHESIS
*INTERVERTEBRAL DISK DISPLACEMENT at the subheading, complications
*THORACIC VERTEBRAE

The other terms that have been assigned are these:

CASE REPORT
FEMALE
HIP DISLOCATION with the subheading, radiography
HUMAN
INTERVERTEBRAL DISK DISPLACEMENT with the subheading, radiography
LEG
MIDDLE AGE
MUSCLE SPASTICITY with the subheading, etiology
POSTOPERATIVE COMPLICATIONS
RECURRENCE

These additional assigned terms can be used to find this article on the computer (MEDLINE). It bears repeating that a MeSH heading can often be IM and at other times NIM, depending on whether the idea was one of the main points of the article. Some of the nonstarred (nonasterisked) terms are check tags: CASE REPORT, FEMALE, HUMAN, and MIDDLE AGE.

OTHER BIOMEDICAL ABSTRACTING AND INDEXING SERVICES

So far this chapter has provided an overview of *Index Medicus* and its indexing principles. The next chapter will continue with more on MEDLINE and the other MEDLARS databases. Here, we will resume with other paper indexes. As the librarian, you will need to know what types of information are in many of the abstracting and indexing services. You need also to decide which ones to purchase and/or have accessible for your patrons. You need to know how to search for information in the paper indexes and their various computerized counterparts. After IM the tool to use is *Biological Abstracts* (BA).

BIOLOGICAL ABSTRACTS

BioSciences Information Services (BIOSIS) is the producer of *Biological Abstracts*, or BA. A separately printed publication produced by BIOSIS is *Biolog-*

ical Abstracts/RRM (Reports, Reviews, Meetings). These two sources are often grouped together on the computer and referred to as the BIOSIS Data Base. BIOSIS is the largest index to literature in the life sciences. If that is so, under what circumstances would a librarian or library user consult BIOSIS rather than IM/MEDLINE? The scope of each is somewhat different. If the user is looking for information in research biology or research medicine, both sources serve the purposes very well. It used to be apparent that the choice for clinical medicine was IM over BA. That may be less so now. How about animals? Clearly, BA coverage is much more comprehensive than IM coverage. However, if you are interested in an animal to understand basic biological mechanisms, such as cell division, you will also be well served by IM. With plants, BA is the choice. However, this does take us a little bit away from our topic, biomedicine. In fact, if the plant has a biomedical connection (e.g., it is used as a drug), that literature will be indexed well in IM, too. MEDLINE and BIOSIS do overlap a good bit (Poyer 1984). However, there are many journals that only one of the two cover. If the topic you are concerned with is covered by both indexes, how do you decide which to use? Which do you check first?

DIFFERENCES AND SIMILARITIES OF IM AND BA

Index Medicus and *Biological Abstracts* differ greatly in cost in both print and computer. A subscription to IM is about $250 and the annual *Cumulated Index Medicus* is around $300. *Biological Abstracts* with its annual indexes is over $7,000. Subscribing to *Biological Abstracts/RRM* with indexes adds another $3,000. The cost to search online on MEDLINE is about $20 per hour. The charge for BIOSIS will be higher. The higher cost of BIOSIS is now due to the much higher citation charges (i.e., over $1.00 per citation displayed). How much does it cost to lease the CD-ROMs? These charges may be expected to change greatly over time and with various vendors and agreements. However, it would be a surprise if BIOSIS were not substantially more than MEDLINE. If you are considering only price, IM/MEDLINE is the clear choice.

Biological Abstracts contains abstracts (*Biological Abstracts/RRM* does not), whereas IM has none. However, since the mid-1970s, MEDLINE has contained author-written abstracts for a growing percentage of its records. Therefore if you want to be sure to get an abstract and, in some cases written by someone other than the author, BA is the choice. *Biological Abstracts* is the best choice if limited to the paper product. In your search, do you want to include sources of information in addition to the journal articles? *Biological Abstracts/RRM* contains book chapters, technical reports, and papers presented at meetings. Except for a brief period in the 1970s when it included some book chapters, IM lists exclusively journal articles. Unless you want to limit your search to journals, BIOSIS is the choice.

Do you feel the need to get the most recently published material? Is a one-to three-month delay too long? Well, you may need to go to sources beyond IM and BA. Other sources may be faster. For some journals, IM may have just one or two months' lag time from publication of the journal to appearance in IM. Online access may present occasions when the elapsed time is less than a month now that the additions to the database are more frequent than once per month. However, the inclusion of the abstracts has always added time to the preparation. The lag time for both BIOSIS and MEDLINE has been getting shorter over the years.

In your selection of databases to search, there are different ways you may look at their journal coverages. MEDLINE is currently expanding its number of journals. Yet, BIOSIS covers a larger number of sources than MEDLINE. Which covers more or fewer journals on the topic you are looking for? Compare the lists of the journals covered by MEDLINE and BIOSIS. Sometimes, the one with more sources may not be the one you choose. You may want to limit your retrieval to the more select or prestigious group of journals. For journals covered by both IM and BA, remember another point. Most of the journals are not indexed cover to cover, and IM and BA may not select the same articles for indexing. If you are seeking comprehensiveness, search both. Overall, remember that there are a number of journals that are in one but not in the other.

The next difference concerns the method of accessing the information—the structure of the index(es). Structure may determine which service you use, BA or IM. *Index Medicus* has one author index and one subject index. *Biological Abstracts* has one author index and three subject indexes (four subject indexes on the computer).

THE INDEXES OF BA

The BA author index is similar to the IM author index in that it uses only initials for the first and middle names, which are placed after the last name without a comma. Here are a few entries for authors in volume 93, January–June 1992, one in the *B*'s and one in the *G*'s.

BROOK I	10641	18068
	18251	37935
GRANT E G	12043	26222
		70843

Which would you rather use? For BA, you need to look up the author and then go to the abstract number that has the citation. This example with Brook and Grant contains just three or four numbers to check in the abstracts section, but you would need to check all the numbers until you found the article you wanted. In addition, BA comes out twice as often—two per month—as IM and the cumulated index is issued twice per year instead of once per year. Along with that, a number of authors are so prolific that they have a dozen or more articles indexed each six months. Therefore, if you were looking for a paper written in mid-1991, you might need to check the January–June 1991 index, the July–December 1991 index, the January–June 1992 index, and perhaps even the July–December 1992 index. With IM, check the cumulation for 1991 and for 1992. The citation will be right there in the author index if you are looking under the first author of the article. *Index Medicus*'s author index is faster to use. Going back to BA, let's say that the citation that we needed is 12043. The abstracts are arranged in numerical order starting with number 1 in the first January issue and then again in the first July issue. This abstract number takes us to the January 1, 1992 issue, volume 93, no. 1. Here is what we find at 12043.

12043. KIMME-SMITH, CAROLYN, RITA R. PERRELLA, LASZLO P. KAVEGGIA, SACHIKO COCHRAN AND EDWARD G. GRANT. (Dep. Radiology, University California Los Angeles, School Medicine, Los Angeles, Calif. 90024.) AJR (AM J ROENTGENOL) 157(5): 975–980. 1991. Detection of renal stones with real-time sonography: Effect of transducers and scanning parameters.

After this title follows an abstract of nine sentences. Each semimonthly issue is arranged by broad classifications. This citation is placed under ''Urinary Systems and External Secretions.'' Note also that the authors' first names may be given here, unlike in the author index.

The next index is the biosystematic index. It organizes the entries the way a biologist views the animal and plant kingdoms—phylum, class, order, and family—and not in an alphabetical order. Groups of organisms are together regardless of where they would fall in the alphabet. This organization is reminiscent of the *Tree Structures* of MeSH. One difference is that MeSH orders all its topics hierarchically. *Biological Abstracts* organizes the organisms only in this way. There is no hierarchical arrangement of diseases, for example, as there is in MeSH. Our citation included only human beings, so the biosystematic index has the 12043 entry under ''Hominidae'' and that is subdivided by ''Urinary Pathology.'' This and the following index, generic index, might best be used when interested in animal (but nonhuman) studies. The generic index is arranged in alphabetical order by genus name.

There is another index that BA no longer includes in the paper edition. The index attempted to do for subjects what the Biosystematic Index does for organisms—bring related topics together. As an index in print, it was daunting. It contained hundreds of undifferentiated numbers of abstracts listed under an entry such as ''Cancer Therapy.'' Sometimes a person would take two sets of numbers and compare them for the occurrence of numbers in both lists. This is the postcoordination mentioned earlier, a method best left to machines instead of humans. A computer is much better suited by temperament to do the postcoordinating. And that is where BIOSIS left this index.

THE MAIN SUBJECT INDEX OF BA

Take a close look at Figure 2.2. This is the primary subject index to BA. It may be the strongest reason to use IM instead of BA. Each page has three columns. Each line in a column represents part of a title of an article that is being indexed in that issue or volume. Go to the column on the left. Begin by looking at the blank space in the middle of a column. Fill in the word RENAL in the blank spaces. The words to the right of the space are in alphabetical order. Follow RENAL down till you get to STONE and then to STONES. Although each of the lines represents the title of an article, it is difficult to read and get the meaning. To the left of the space on a line are the words in the journal article title before that one word. To the right are the words after that word in the title. If you read straight across a line while filling in the blank with the word, you will have part of the title. Only as much of the title that fits into a column width is there, and the slash mark (/) shows the beginning of a title. To find the full title, you do the same thing you did with the other indexes: Take the number to the right, the abstract number, and consult the full record. This example, ''N METHOD/DETECTION OF RENAL STONES WITH REAL-TIME SONOGRAP'' is understandable. Well, at least it is coherent. Sometimes it is difficult to decipher the meaning from these shortened, chopped-up titles. Another title near the top of that column (second line) displays this: NIST BLOCKS ANP-INDUCED RENAL RESPONSES THROUGH A SPECIFIC I (138371). The full article title from that entry is ''HS-142–1, a novel nonpeptide atrial natriuretic peptide (ANP) antagonist, blocks ANP-induced renal responses through a specific interaction with guanylyl cyclase-linked receptors.'' The segments given in this index are the same length regardless of title length. Four points should be noted about the words in this index: (1) the words are taken from the author's title and are presented in that order; (2) BIOSIS adds other words to the end of the title to augment the retrieval; (3) only as much of the enhanced title that will fit in that space is included; and (4) each non-trivial word of the enhanced title is used as an entry point. Therefore, for the title of the article ''Detection of Renal Stones with Real-Time Sonography: Effect of Transducers and Scanning Parameters,'' there are the following searchable terms:

—renal

—stones

—real-time

—sonography

—transducers

Each of these entry points has the rest of the title portion surrounding it, as we saw with the ''renal'' entry. In BA many words act as indicators of subject content. This is a totally different type of index than used in IM. MeSH is a

Figure 2.2
Primary Subject Index to *Biological Abstracts*

Subject Context	▼ Keyword		Ref. No.
LIVER WEIGHT/ ABNORMAL	**RENAL**	RESPONSE TO TWENTY-FOUR-HOUR D	129538
NIST BLOCKS ANP-INDUCED		RESPONSES THROUGH A SPECIFIC I	138371
TRIURESIS NEPHROPATHY/		RESPONSES TO ACUTE VOLUME EXPA	23676
IBITION POTENTIATES THE		RESPONSES TO NEUTRAL ENDOPEPTI	13917
FFECTS OF NIFEDIPINE ON		RESPONSES TO SEVERAL DIURETIC	11923
IAL NATRIURETIC PEPTIDE		RESPONSES VASODILATION/ EFFECT	91696
EM/ CAPTOPRIL ENHANCES		RESPONSIVENESS TO ANF IN DOGS	138369
ABSORPTION BONE RELEASE		RETENTION NEUROTOXIC IMPLICATI	30170
TIC RECONSTRUCTION AND		REVASCULARIZATION SAFE AND EFF	25290
RTOGRAPHY PROPHYLACTIC		REVASCULARIZATION/ NATURAL HIS	1762
FECTS HUMAN HEREDITARY		SALT WASHING SYNDROME/ TYPE I	15524
CORD INJURY PATIENTS BY		SCAN TECHNETIUM-99M DIETHYLENE	129577
L PARENCHYMA INFECTION		SCAN/ RELATIONSHIP AMONG VESIC	18060
HY FOR THE DETECTION OF		SCARRING AND ITS CORRELATION W	127259
OTENSIVE CHILDREN WITH		SCARRING ANTIHYPERTENSIVE-DRUG	56444
E RESPONSE HYPERTENSION		SCARRING ETIOLOGY/ CAPTOPRIL T	94877
/ ANTIOXIDANT EFFECT ON		SCARRING FOLLOWING INFECTION O	89352
OSIS OF POST-INFECTIOUS		SCARRING IN RELATION TO RADIOL	89493
G VESICOURETERIC REFLEX		SCARRING METHOD/ IMAGING IN U	42013
TIS PREVENTION POSSIBLE		SCARRING PREVENTION TEST SENSI	118381
IA-COLI STRAINS CAUSING		SCARRING PYELONEPHRITIS/ EXTRA	18245
ON IN THE MINIATURE PIG		SCARRING RENAL ISCHEMIA PATHOG	83692
W UP CHILD RENAL LENGTH		SCARRING UROGRAPHY TREATMENT/	41957
METHOD/ EVALUATION OF		SCARS BY TECHNETIUM-LABELED DI	118383
PHY DOPPLER SONOGRAPHY		SCINTIGRAPHY ANGIOGRAPHY SCREE	1864
RIA CYSTOURETHROGRAPHY		SCINTIGRAPHY RADIONUCLIDE CYST	106730
TERIZED TOMOGRAPHY AND		SELECTIVE ANGIOGRAPHY IN PREOP	66819
LASMA PROTEIN BINDING/		SELECTIVE N ACETYL-L-GAMMA-GLU	32293
THOPHYSIOLOGY/ NORMAL		SENSITIVITY TO ATRIAL NATRIURE	85228
ANDINS IN ACTIVATION OF		SENSORY RECEPTORS RAT PROSTAGL	72182
ASOUND LOCALIZATION FOR		SHIELDING HUMAN RADIOTHERAPY	19372
MAL TUBULE/ MUZOLIMINE		SITE OF ACTION AND INTERACTION	45024
TION/ EVALUATION OF THE		SITE OF ACTION OF A NOVEL EUKA	103712
VOUS SYSTEM CYCLIC GMP/		SITES OF ACTION OF PHYSIOLOGIC	96514
RODILATIN IN CONTROL OF		SODIUM EXCRETION DOG CYCLIC GM	140942
NATRIURETIC FACTOR AND		SODIUM EXCRETION DURING VENTIL	120304
UM CHLORIDE LOADS SHEEP		SODIUM EXCRETION LAMINA TERMI	83737
ATRIURETIC FACTOR LEVEL		SODIUM EXCRETION/ DIETARY SODI	49359
ND HYPERTENSION HUMAN		SODIUM HANDLING ALTERATION/ PL	1799
XCRETION IN RELATION TO		SODIUM HANDLING IN MINIMAL CH	47626
NISM/ EXPRESSION OF RAT		SODIUM PHOSPHATE COTRANSPORTE	129618
/ MOLECULAR SIZE OF THE		SODIUM PHOSPHATE SYMPORTER IN	129619
M-3 GD-3 ON THE PORCINE		SODIUM POTASSIUM ATPASE ACTIVI	118391
ON/ CHARACTERIZATION OF		SODIUM POTASSIUM ATPASE GENE E	118390
ROTATIONAL DYNAMICS OF		SODIUM POTASSIUM ATPASE STUDIE	126435
ISTRIBUTION OF A RABBIT		SODIUM PROTON EXCHANGER TRANS	64324
MERULAR FILTRATION RATE		SODIUM TRANSPORT PATHOPHYSIOL	72106
TING PHARMACOKINETICS/		SPECIFIC DELIVERY OF SULFAMETH	120380
ORN LAMBS BARORECEPTOR		STIMULUS-RESPONSE CURVE/ PLASM	140930
TED PYELONEPHRITIS WITH		STONE A PROPOSED INDEX OF LOCA	25669
EDAP LT-01 HUMAN URETER		STONE ANALGESIA NEED/ OUTPATIE	83662
CONCENTRATING CAPACITY		STONE DISEASE RENAL CALCULI OS	15672
RIZOATE DIAGNOSTIC-DRUG		STONE DISEASE UROGRAPHY/ USE O	92443
ITHIASIS DRUG TREATMENT		STONE FORMATION INFECTED NEPHR	12036
IHYDRATE METHYLENE BLUE		STONE FORMATION X-RAY POWDER	129565
PROCESSES REVIEW HUMAN		STONE FORMATION/ THE ROLE OF T	129567
RATHYROIDECTOMY HUMAN		STONE GLOMERULAR FILTRATION RA	63672
OSITION IN CONTROLS AND		STONE PATIENTS FROM NORTHEASTE	34546
RINARY ACIDIFICATION IN		STONE PATIENTS FROM NORTHEASTE	105308
D CYSTINE STONES HUMAN		STONE STONE IMPACTION CATHETER	59812
MY IN SELECTED PATIENTS		STONE THERAPEUTIC METHOD/ SHO	140871
ACTING-DRUG RENAL COLIC		STONE ULTRASOUND PERISTALSIS U	115816
RPARATHYROIDISM HUMAN		STONE/ CONSERVATIVE MANAGEMEN	15673
IDANCE RENAL PATHOLOGY		STONE/ ENDOLUMINAL UROLOGIC UL	11999
UM PHOSPHATES OXALATES		STONES CLINICAL PROFILE BIOCHE	59840
HATE IN CALCIUM OXALATE		STONES HUMAN ANALYTICAL METHO	106768
IC DIETARY TREATMENT IN		STONES HUMAN CALCIUM RECURREN	59810
OCCUPATIONAL EXPOSURE		STONES HYPEROXALURIA GASTROINT	129562
ARY TRACT CALCULI HUMAN		STONES URETERAL STONES FRAGMEN	118334
EASE HUMAN UROLITHIASIS		STONES URETERIC STONES/ FAMILY	72100
N METHOD/ DETECTION OF		STONES WITH REAL-TIME SONOGRAP	12043
F AMMONIA TRANSPORT IN		STRAIGHT PROXIMAL TUBULES MOUS	36013
HOLOGY HISTOCHEMISTRY/		STRUCTURAL CHANGES IN MYOCARD	35935
-INDUCED ALTERATIONS IN		STRUCTURE AMMONIAGENESIS AND	72154
IHYPERTENSIVE TOXICITY/		STRUCTURE AND FUNCTION IN RATS	83592
ATHY AND IMPAIRMENT OF		STRUCTURES HUMAN T CELL B CELL	23709
PAROTOMY/ SPONTANEOUS		SUBCAPSULAR HEMATOMA AN UNUS	23726
SLETS TRANSPLANTED INTO		SUBCAPSULAR SPACE DIABETES IMM	75667
TINUOUS EXTRACORPOREAL		SUPPORT IN PAEDIATRIC INTENSIV	23722
N FAILURE HUMAN UREMIA		SUPPORT METHOD HEMODIALYSIS/	59823
TECTION IN PERCUTANEOUS		SURGERY HUMAN ENDOSCOPIC SURG	128530
REACTIVE OXYGEN SPECIES		SYMPATHETIC ACTIVATION MORPHO	96532
EAGLE ARTERIAL PRESSURE		SYMPATHETIC ACTIVITY HEMODYNA	31334
EFFECT OF YOHIMBINE ON		SYMPATHETIC NERVE ACTIVITY AND	102602
USTAINED SUPPRESSION OF		SYMPATHETIC NERVE ACTIVITY BY	74080
SODIUM CHLORIDE INTAKE		SYMPATHETIC NERVE ACTIVITY HEA	73700
TUS SOLITARII INCREASED		SYMPATHETIC NERVE ACTIVITY HYP	119797
OREFLEX SYSTEM/ ROLE OF		SYMPATHETIC NERVE ACTIVITY IN	25226
FUNDAMENTAL RHYTHM OF		SYMPATHETIC NERVE ACTIVITY IN	125861
N ON THE PERIODICITY OF		SYMPATHETIC NERVE ACTIVITY IN	125870
DE SYNTHESIS STIMULATES		SYMPATHETIC NERVE ACTIVITY IN-	120180
TS ON HEMODYNAMICS AND		SYMPATHETIC NERVE ACTIVITY RAT	56821
ESSURE MUSCLE PARALYSIS		SYMPATHETIC NERVE ACTIVITY REN	137045
KIDNEYS NOREPINEPHRINE		SYMPATHETIC NERVE ACTIVITY/ SE	140853
OUS PRESSURE HEART RATE		SYMPATHETIC NERVE RENAL VASCUL	36014
C FACTOR BIRTH/ ROLE OF		SYMPATHETIC NERVES IN LAMBS DU	55823
OF ADRENAL SPLENIC AND		SYMPATHETIC NERVES IN THE RAT	55987
RIAL NATRIURETIC FACTOR		SYMPATHETIC NERVES MEAN ARTERI	12151
PECTRAL ANALYSIS OF THE		SYMPATHETIC NEUROGRAM DURING	13714
AEMORRHAGIC FEVER WITH		SYNDROME ARBOVIRUS HUMAN HEM	89578
HEMORRHAGIC FEVER WITH		SYNDROME BY A NEUTRALIZATION T	82395
HEMORRHAGIC FEVER WITH		SYNDROME COMPARISON OF CLINIC	66307
HEMORRHAGIC FEVER WITH		SYNDROME HUMAN ANTIVIRAL-DRUG	34417
AEMORRHAGIC FEVER WITH		SYNDROME HUMAN HANTAAN VIRUS	78304
HEMORRHAGIC FEVER WITH		SYNDROME PATHOGENESIS DENSE P	89578
HEMORRHAGIC FEVER WITH		SYNDROME VIRUS HEP-2 CELLS WIS	83781
HEMORRHAGIC FEVER WITH		SYNDROME VIRUS HUMAN TOTAL T C	17312
HEMORRHAGIC FEVER WITH		SYNDROME VIRUS HUMAN URINE CE	78378
HEMORRHAGIC FEVER WITH		SYNDROME VIRUS IN LYMPHOCYTE S	42142
AEMORRHAGIC FEVER WITH		SYNDROME VIRUS INFECTION ARBOV	17312
OGRAPHY/ A STUDY ON THE		SYNTHESIS OF DOPAMINE IN AGED	36010
ITERATURE REVIEW HUMAN		SYSTEM HEART CENTRAL NERVOUS S	74781
OSTAGLANDIN SYNTHESIS/		SYSTEMS REGULATING WATER-ELECT	23791
NCER DIAGNOSTIC METHOD		TIME SCANNER MECHANICAL ARC SC	113416
BETA-2 MICROGLOBULIN IN		TISSUE AS AN INDICATOR OF RENA	106736
MODEL BIOACCUMULATION		TISSUE CONCENTRATION PLASMA CO	23588
JC VIRUS DNA IN NORMAL		TISSUE DERIVED FROM TUMOR-BEAR	94968
CLEARANCE/ URINARY AND		TISSUE INSULIN-LIKE GROWTH FAC	12014
N HUMAN SPLANCHNIC AND		TISSUES BLOOD FLOW BLOOD PRESS	25524
DOTA EVALUATION OF ITS		TOLERANCE IN PATIENTS WITH CHR	103701
ETIC RESONANCE IMAGING/		TOLERANCE OF AMI 25 RAT DIAGNO	59707
ETIC RESONANCE IMAGING/		TOLERANCE OF GADOLINIUM DTPA D	106752
INC PRETREATMENT ON THE		TOXICITY AND INTRARENAL ACCUMU	83264
IDE ANTINEOPLASTIC-DRUG		TOXICITY ANTIDOTE-DRUG/ A FEAS	43144
ROGEN MYELOSUPPRESSION		TOXICITY BONE SOFT TISSUE/ CHE	19261
ICOLOGY PATHOGENIC DIET		TOXICITY GASTROINTESTINAL TOXI	59442
OLE OF CHELATORS RABBIT		TOXICITY HEAVY METAL/ NATURE O	35677
FOLLOW-UP OF IFOSFAMIDE		TOXICITY IN CHILDREN TREATED F	43193
E NAG FOR EVALUATION OF		TOXICITY INDUCED BY CHEMOTHERA	42970
EPATIC METALLOTHIONEIN		TOXICITY METAL CHELATION/ TIME	23257
BINDING HEPATIC FAILURE		TOXICITY MINIMUM INHIBITORY CO	74224
WITH ANION-GAP ACIDOSIS		TOXICITY NMR DIAGNOSTIC METHO	47354
ENT PHARMACODYNAMICS/		TOXICITY OF ENALAPRIL IN VERY	47572
ANTITUMOR ACTIVITY AND		TOXICITY OF THE LATTER IN NUDE	31231
ON CIS PLATINUM-INDUCED		TOXICITY RAT FOSFOMYCIN ANTINE	67028
DRUG PHARMACODYNAMICS		TOXICITY WEIGHT LOSS/ OPTIMAL	67205
CCHAROMYCES-CEREVISIAE		TOXICITY 2 3 BISPHOSPHOGLYCERA	135379
TS HUMAN TOXICOKINETICS		TOXICITY/ IBUPROFEN OVERDOSE I	129462
ISEASE HEPATIC TOXICITY		TOXICITY/ LOW-DOSE AMPHOTERICI	38007
IOR HUMAN ANIMAL MODEL	**RENAL**	TOXICOLOGY NEUROTOXICOLOGY CO	35684
GS ANTINEOPLASTIC AGENT		TOXICOSIS/ EFFECT OF TIME OF C	23572
RIGLYCINE IN PAEDIATRIC		TRACT DISEASE CHILD PEDIATRICS	81328
MAN PRENATAL DIAGNOSIS		TRACT MALFORMATIONS OLIGOHYDR	14753
HOD/ THE MANAGEMENT OF		TRANSPLANT ARTERY STENOSIS IN	131070
INE MATHEMATICAL MODEL		TRANSPLANT DONOR TECHNETIUM-9	59870
NT ACUTE NEPHROTOXICITY		TRANSPLANT GLOMERULAR FILTRATI	11926
UMAN CIRCADIAN RHYTHM		TRANSPLANT HEMODIALYSIS PERITO	106733
FUSION REVISITED HUMAN		TRANSPLANT HLA ALLOGRAFT SURVI	1361
DELAYED GRAFT FUNCTION		TRANSPLANT MEDICARE HEALTH CAR	10604
ISCHEMIC HEART DISEASE		TRANSPLANT MORTALITY SURVIVAL	8533
IVE WOUND INFECTIONS IN		TRANSPLANT PATIENTS A MATCHED-	135383
ICS OF CYCLOSPORIN A IN		TRANSPLANT PATIENTS AFTER INFU	32808
INE PHARMACOKINETICS IN		TRANSPLANT PATIENTS ANTIHYPERT	44670
ANTIBODIES IN SERUM OF		TRANSPLANT PATIENTS HUMAN CYTO	134658
ACTIN ON CYCLOSPORIN IN		TRANSPLANT PATIENTS HUMAN IMM	115412
IDIOTYPES ANTIBODIES IN		TRANSPLANT PATIENTS REVIEW HU	65260
SUPPRESSANT-DRUG LIVER		TRANSPLANT RADIOIMMUNOASSAY	68772
S EPIDIDYMO-ORCHITIS IN		TRANSPLANT RECIPIENT CASE REPO	35790
D KAPOSI'S SARCOMA IN A		TRANSPLANT RECIPIENT HUMAN IM	6908
S ANTIBODY SEROPOSITIVE		TRANSPLANT RECIPIENT TREATED W	89570
ASPHYXIA/ PREGNANCY IN		TRANSPLANT RECIPIENTS CASE REP	82752
IN CYCLOSPORINE-TREATED		TRANSPLANT RECIPIENTS HUMAN CG	103405
IN ON HYPERLIPIDEMIA IN		TRANSPLANT RECIPIENTS HUMAN EN	91866
IALYSIS/ HEPATITIS C IN		TRANSPLANT RECIPIENTS HUMAN HE	54206
STAGE RENAL FAILURE AND		TRANSPLANT RECIPIENTS HUMAN HO	29920
ETIC FACTOR INFUSION IN		TRANSPLANT RECIPIENTS HUMAN HO	103705
OMEGALOVIRUS DISEASE IN		TRANSPLANT RECIPIENTS HUMAN HY	25773
YPERLIPIDEMIA IN STABLE		TRANSPLANT RECIPIENTS HUMAN PL	12050
AFT SURVIVAL IN CADAVER		TRANSPLANT RECIPIENTS HUMAN PR	94816
TERLEUKIN 2 RECEPTOR IN		TRANSPLANT RECIPIENTS HUMAN RE	94814
DISEASE AND SURVIVAL IN		TRANSPLANT RECIPIENTS/ THE IMP	89572
OF THE UNOS SCIENTIFIC		TRANSPLANT REGISTRY AT THREE Y	83979
PLER DIAGNOSIS OF ACUTE		TRANSPLANT REJECTION HUMAN DIA	77286
N PATIENTS WITH CHRONIC		TRANSPLANT REJECTION HUMAN PLA	83652
MMUNOSUPPRESSANT-DRUG		TRANSPLANT REJECTION/ EFFECTS	20944
EMIA IN RECIPIENTS OF A		TRANSPLANT WHO ARE TREATED WI	106673
NT-DRUG RENAL DISORDER		TRANSPLANT/ EFFECTS OF DEFIBRO	9221
IGHT-GIEMSA CASE REPORT		TRANSPLANT/ MORPHOLOGICAL DIA	101105
SSANT-DRUG SIDE EFFECTS		TRANSPLANTATION ALLOGRAFT REJE	92071
SMA FLOW RPF FOLLOWING		TRANSPLANTATION BY USE OF FUNC	35999
OURETERAL REFLUX IN THE		TRANSPLANTATION CANDIDATE HUM	29982
RAWAL OF STEROIDS AFTER		TRANSPLANTATION CLINICAL PREDI	92067
N KIDNEY CELLS IN-VITRO		TRANSPLANTATION COMPLICATION H	6264
TIAL FUNCTION FOLLOWING		TRANSPLANTATION DETERMINED BY	56759
ETERAL STRICTURES AFTER		TRANSPLANTATION DIAGNOSIS AND	59816
CITY/ PROTEINURIA AFTER		TRANSPLANTATION DIAGNOSIS WIT	47634
D OUTCOME OF CADAVERIC		TRANSPLANTATION DUE TO CALCIUM	11975
LYSIS PATIENTS AWAITING		TRANSPLANTATION END STAGE RENA	94857
DYNAMICS MODEL HUMAN		TRANSPLANTATION EPIDEMIOLOGY/	70702
TE GRAFT SURVIVAL RATE/		TRANSPLANTATION FOR SYSTEMIC L	53331
FT SURVIVAL STATISTICS/		TRANSPLANTATION FROM HLA-HAPLO	140834
ALPORT'S SYNDROME AFTER		TRANSPLANTATION GRAFT ANTIGLO	53333
AL REPLACEMENT THERAPY		TRANSPLANTATION HEMODIALYSIS C	78402
CR AMPLIFICATION HUMAN		TRANSPLANTATION HISTOCOMPATIB	123452
GROWTH HORMONE AFTER		TRANSPLANTATION HORMONE-DRUG	87035
OUTCOME AFTER CADAVER		TRANSPLANTATION HUMAN CARDIOV	44247
TE CHOLINE UPTAKE AFTER		TRANSPLANTATION HUMAN CREATIN	83694
RONIC RENAL FAILURE AND		TRANSPLANTATION HUMAN CYCLOSP	53332
L STUDIES WITH FK506 IN		TRANSPLANTATION HUMAN CYCLOSP	92082
UPPRESSION IN CADAVERIC		TRANSPLANTATION HUMAN CYTOME	134545
N DURING ANESTHESIA FOR		TRANSPLANTATION HUMAN ENZYME	8677
ATIONS IN SERUM DURING		TRANSPLANTATION HUMAN GENERAL	92275
LUDING CYCLOSPORINE FOR		TRANSPLANTATION HUMAN IMMUNO	115389
IS AND AFTER SUCCESSFUL		TRANSPLANTATION HUMAN LUTEINIZ	58727
OMPLICATIONS FOLLOWING		TRANSPLANTATION HUMAN MORBIDI	34528
ATIVE BACILLI FOLLOWING		TRANSPLANTATION HUMAN PNEUMO	29975
ENITAL MALIGNANCIES AND		TRANSPLANTATION HUMAN REJECTI	89798
RENAL FAILURE AND AFTER		TRANSPLANTATION IMPACT ON HYPE	140831
ND STAGE RENAL DISEASE/		TRANSPLANTATION IN CHILDREN WI	47649
INO-9-BENZYLGUANINE ON		TRANSPLANTATION IN DOG ENZYME	8829
TIC SYNDROME FOLLOWING		TRANSPLANTATION IN PATIENTS WI	53334
ND STAGE RENAL DISEASE/		TRANSPLANTATION IN PATIENTS 65	140866
PAEDIATRIC DIALYSIS AND		TRANSPLANTATION IN THE STATE R	94882
EPHROPATHIC CYSTINOSIS/		TRANSPLANTATION IN 22 CHILDREN	72119
EOPERATIVE ASSESSMENT/		TRANSPLANTATION INTO ABNORMAL	47656
ACUTE TUBULAR NECROSIS		TRANSPLANTATION ISCHEMIA/ PROT	81317
-DRUG PHARMACOKINETICS		TRANSPLANTATION MATHEMATICAL	44624
MMUNOCOMPETENCE/ POST		TRANSPLANTATION NON-HODGKIN'S	113234
G-TERM COMPLICATIONS OF		TRANSPLANTATION REVIEW HUMAN	83647
EUTIC METHOD/ PEDIATRIC		TRANSPLANTATION REVIEW HUMAN	137523
HYLAXIS OF INFECTION IN		TRANSPLANTATION SIDE EFFECTS O	62085
BERTAL GROWTH DIAL`'IS		TRANSPLANTATION TANNER GENITAL	12029
RENAL HYPOTHERMIA DOG		TRANSPLANTATION THERAPEUTIC M	72076
MUNOSUPPRESSANT AGENT		TRANSPLANTATION UVEITIS/ USEFU	118254
ENCE OF INFECTION AFTER		TRANSPLANTATION WITH THE USE O	81006
ISEASE MORTALITY SEPSIS		TRANSPLANTATION/ ACUTE RENAL F	35979
KIN-7 INTERFERON-GAMMA		TRANSPLANTATION/ CYTOKINE AND	88591
DRUG-DRUG INTERACTION		TRANSPLANTATION/ DIAGNOSIS OF	56717
GLOBULIN G ANTIIDIOTYPE		TRANSPLANTATION/ PREDICTION OF	92070
GLUTATHIONE COENZYME A		TRANSPLANTATION/ PROTECTIVE EF	35990
H CHRONIC RENAL FAILURE		TRANSPLANTS AND PERIODONTITIS	54104
N ZERO-HOUR BIOPSIES OF		TRANSPLANTS HUMAN AGE DEPENDE	47624
SONANCE ANGIOGRAPHY OF		TRANSPLANTS HUMAN ARTERIAL STE	131128
IN CHRONICALLY REJECTED		TRANSPLANTS HUMAN END-STAGE RE	100259
FUNCTION OR OUTCOME OF		TRANSPLANTS HUMAN MAJOR HISTO	123468
E LEVELS/ SONOGRAPHY OF		TRANSPLANTS IN DOGS THE EFFECT	123680
RESSANT-DRUG/ PEDIATRIC		TRANSPLANTS RESULTS WITH SEQUE	92068
T FUNCTION IN CADAVERIC		TRANSPLANTS TREATED WITH LOW	68760
PATHOLOGIC FEATURES OF		TRANSPLANTS WITH ANTI-CLASS I-	134549
N PROXIMAL NEPHRON AND		TRANSPORT PHARMACOLOGICAL TOO	36003
UBULAR LUMEN SECRETION		TRANSPORT SYSTEM VIDEO IMAGING	72200
L INTERVENTION IN BLUNT		TRAUMA HUMAN DIAGNOSTIC METH	140864
HIC ASSESSMENT OF BLUNT		TRAUMA HUMAN RENAL CONTUSIONS	47635
EATMENT OF 429 CASES OF		TRAUMA HUMAN RENAL LESIONS CO	22528
TIVE DECISION-MAKING IN		TRAUMA SURGERY HUMAN HEMORRH	35921
S FIBRINOUS THROMBOSIS		TUBE SIDEROSIS HEPATIC CHOLEST	79063
IA FEVER PRENATAL CARE/		TUBERCULOSIS AND PREGNANCY A C	18002
OMA DIAGNOSTIC METHOD/		TUBERCULOSIS DIAGNOSIS WITH SO	124187
ATIENTS WITH CAVERNOUS		TUBERCULOSIS IMMUNOLOGIC-DRUG	18331
ENTAL AMALGAM IMPAIRED		TUBULAR ABSORPTION/ MERCURY F	11801
TARY DNA OSTEOPETROSIS		TUBULAR ACIDOSIS CEREBRAL CALC	111473
USES HYPOKALEMIC DISTAL		TUBULAR ACIDOSIS RAT COLLECTIN	140854
IN II HUMAN HYPOKALEMIA		TUBULAR ACIDOSIS/ SELECTIVE HY	12055
IURESIS DIURESIS/ ACUTE		TUBULAR AND HEMODYNAMIC EFFEC	44244
-KININ RECEPTORS IN THE		TUBULAR AND HEMODYNAMIC RESPO	83744
PROTON EXCHANGE IN RAT		TUBULAR BRUSH-BORDER MEMBRAN	72194
RYSTALS WITH A CULTURED		TUBULAR CELL LINE CANINE HUMAN	12048
ERICIN B AGAINST RABBIT		TUBULAR CELLS IN PRIMARY CULTU	74259
ES ADHESION TO CULTURED		TUBULAR CELLS PORCINE LLC-PK-1	66030
SEASES PANCREATIC RNASE		TUBULAR DAMAGE PANCREATITIS/ U	120932
H EXCRETION IN CHRONIC		TUBULAR DISORDERS COMPARISON	12040
APID IMPROVEMENT IN THE		TUBULAR DYSFUNCTION ASSOCIATED	94869
RETINOL-BINDING PROTEIN		TUBULAR DYSFUNCTION DIABETIC N	23747
L INJURY RAT CREATININE		TUBULAR DYSFUNCTION GLOMERULO	47664
NSIN CONVERTING ENZYME		TUBULAR DYSGENESIS FETAL HYPOT	2699
SSENGER RNA EXPRESSION/		TUBULAR EPITHELIAL CELLS EXPRE	72222
OCCUS-SAPROPHYTICUS TO		TUBULAR EPITHELIAL CELLS IS ME	18197
E FOR IRON ANIMAL ACUTE		TUBULAR EPITHELIAL INJURY/ HYD	11806
TERIZATION OF CDNA FROM		TUBULAR EPITHELIUM ENCODING M	72230
AND REACTIVATION IS THE		TUBULAR EPITHELIUM POLYOMAVIR	54283
AL VASODILATOR RESPONSE		TUBULAR FUNCTION LOCAL BLOOD F	72218
LACTATE DEHYDROGENASE		TUBULAR FUNCTION POLYURIA TUBU	118319
ALCAEMIA HEMODYNAMICS		TUBULAR FUNCTION RENOTROPIC FA	113526
NEYS PHARMACOKINETICS/		TUBULAR HANDLING OF P AMINOHIP	91936
H TWO FORMS OF PRIMARY		TUBULAR HYPOKALEMIC ALKALOSIS	66366
CASES HUMAN OSTEOBLAST		TUBULAR INVESTIGATION PATHOPHY	1469
YTE PULMONARY ALVEOLUS		TUBULAR LUMINA ADRENAL CORTICA	135517
STIC AID/ ESTIMATION OF		TUBULAR SECRETION IN MAN IN HE	59783
DEVELOPMENT/ INCREASED	**RENAL**	TUBULAR SODIUM POTASSIUM ATPA	61571
S AT RISK OF DEVELOPING		TUBULAR TOXICITY ASSOCIATED WI	67296
AL ENZYME INDUCTORS ON		TUBULAR TRANSPORT OF IODAMIDE	91899
TIVE TUBULAR SECRETION/		TUBULAR TRANSPORT OF MORPHINE	33043
CONTRAST MEDIA-INDUCED		TUBULAR VACUOLIZATION A LIGHT	59708
CONTRAST MEDIA-INDUCED		TUBULAR VACUOLIZATION AFTER DE	106638
R TRANSPORT IN THE NEWT		TUBULE DUE TO THE ACTION OF LO	129616
IN DEFINED CULTURES OF		TUBULE EPITHELIA A ROLE FOR CY	94698
SIONS IN THE SPLEEN AND		TUBULE EPITHELIA OF TURKEYS AN	112970
RE OF THE ELASMOBRANCH		TUBULE INTERMEDIATE DISTAL AND	59775
EPITHELIAL HEP-2 CELLS		TUBULE LLC-PK-1 CELLS HEMOLYSI	124264
T ANTIDIURETIC HORMONE		TUBULE OSMOSIS GRAVIMETRIC MET	23767
OLUME EXPANSION IN RATS		TUBULE RENAL PLASMA FLOW GLOME	114577
YL AMMONIUM TRANSPORT		TUBULE SECRETION PH SENSITIVIT	36028
F UREA TRANSPORT ACROSS		TUBULES BY PYRAZINOYLGUANIDINE	138373
SUCCINYLACETONE IN RAT		TUBULES FERROCHELATASE HEME OX	59903
GREGATION LITHOGENESIS		TUBULES LUMEN/ PHYSICO-CHEMICA	12033
ETION IN ISOLATED SNAKE		TUBULES P AMINOHIPPURATE ALPHA	36036
RALICHTHYS-LETHOSTIGMA		TUBULES RAT CRAB SOUTHERN FLOU	72200
IUM OXALATE CRYSTALS IN		TUBULES RAT URINARY STONE DISE	129566
NCE FIMBRIAL BINDING TO		TUBULI AND IMMOBILIZED FIBRONE	78030
ULTRASONIC DIAGNOSIS OF		TUMOR AN ANALYSIS OF 82 CASES	18951
HUMAN PROSTATIC TUMOR		TUMOR BLADDER TUMOR NEW OPER	34131
IQUES HUMAN RENAL CYST		TUMOR CORTICAL SCARRING COLUM	83707
IN CYCLOSPORINE-INDUCED		TUMOR FROM DIABETIC RATS BIOPT	6496
UCOCORTICOID RECEPTORS		TUMOR/ HORMONE RECEPTORS STUD	19068
OMA BONE METASTASIZING		TUMOR/ TAMM-HORSFALL PROTEIN I	89818
S' AND OTHER CHILDHOOD		TUMORS NEPHROBLASTOMA HYPERD	19144
AND CHEMICALLY INDUCED		TUMORS OF THE RAT N NITROSODIM	66658
CONSERVATIVE SURGERY OF		TUMORS SURGICAL TECHNIQUE COM	79273
CONSERVATIVELY RESECTED		TUMORS USING AUTOMATED IMAGE	7226
RING TUMOR DEVELOPMENT		TUMORS/ HIGH SUSCEPTIBILITY OF	101540
ARIAN PROSTATE BLADDER		TUMORS/ IMMUNOHISTOCHEMICAL	6878
RECEPTORS STUDIES WITH		TUMOURS MEDROXYPROGESTERONE	19068
RSFALL PROTEIN IN HUMAN		TUMOURS RHABDOID KIDNEY TUMO	89818
ODUCT P21 IN CHILDHOOD		TUMOURS TUMOR IMMUNOPEROXID	42356
L FAILURE BY INCREASING		TXA-2 SYNTHESIS IN RAT? ANTIBI	140703
NTHRENE ON HEPATIC AND		T4 METABOLISM AND THYROID GLAN	42465
CINOMA/ INTRAOPERATIVE		ULTRASONOGRAPHY A USEFUL ADJU	19529
F URINARY DRAINAGE IN A		UNIT WITH AN INDWELLING DOUBLE	23677
AND SEX DIFFERENCES IN		UPTAKE OF METHYLMERCURY IN MIC	35757
ERTENSION/ DIFFERENTIAL		UPTAKE OF THALLIUM-201 REQUIRE	12098
ION LITHOTRIPTOR HUMAN		URETERAL STONE FRAGMENTATION S	83661
OSTAGLANDIN SYSTEMS IN		URIC ACID METABOLISM IN PATIEN	73717
LIURESIS/ IMPAIRMENT OF		URINARY EXCRETION IN NEONATAL	94672
MAN ANTIBACTERIAL-DRUG		URINARY EXCRETION/ AN OPEN STU	37967
G FACTOR IN THE IN-VIVO		VASCULAR ACTION OF ADENOSINE I	120229
UM IN HYPERTENSIVE RATS		VASCULAR CHANGES/ DEUTERIUM O	1776
NSLUMINAL ANGIOPLASTY/		VASCULAR HYPERTENSION DURING P	10813
YCORTICOSTERONE SALT OR		VASCULAR HYPERTENSION GLUCOSE	131052
ENSIVE RAT HYPERTENSION		VASCULAR LESION/ THE EFFECT OF	32056
NCE BETWEEN AORTIC AND		VASCULAR REACTIVITY IN CYCLOSP	140475
CIN PHARMACODYNAMICS/		VASCULAR REACTIVITY TO VASODIL	73798
OUSLY HYPERTENSIVE RATS		VASCULAR REACTIVITY VASODILATO	119841
KALIURESIS NATRIURESIS		VASCULAR RESISTANCE DECREASED	81326
ORT PERFUSATE FLOW RATE		VASCULAR RESISTANCE GLOMERULAR	108880
G IN ANAESTHETIZED RATS		VASCULAR RESISTANCE GLUCOSE ME	129611
ONIC SALINE INFUSION ON		VASCULAR RESISTANCE IN ANESTHE	36014
UG CARDIOVASCULAR-DRUG		VASCULAR RESISTANCE PUTATIVE E	103706
-ARGININE HEMODYNAMICS		VASCULAR RESISTANCE RENAL BLOO	85156
MEAN ARTERIAL PRESSURE		VASCULAR RESISTANCE SYMPATHETI	102660
SIVE-DRUG DIURETIC-DRUG		VASCULAR RESISTANCE/ EFFECT OF	92440
NG-DRUG CARDIAC OUTPUT		VASCULAR RESISTANCE/ RENAL FUN	33219
OLUME RENAL BLOOD FLOW		VASCULAR RESISTANCE/ THE ACUTE	68414
MEAN ARTERIAL PRESSURE		VASCULAR RESISTANCE/ THROMBOX	33225
PHARMACOLOGICAL TOOLS		VASCULAR RESPONSE/ ANALYSIS OF	49695
INCREASED SYSTEMIC AND		VASCULAR SENSITIVITY TO ANGIOT	119839
RENAL SYMPATHETIC NERVE		VASCULAR SMOOTH MUSCLE/ EFFECT	36014
D-LIMB BLOOD FLOW SHEEP		VASCULATURE HEMODYNAMICS PERI	14079
RS IN THE KIDNEY REVIEW		VASCULATURE HYPERTENSION RENAL	59899
AND THROMBOXANE IN RAT		VASCULATURE RECEPTOR AGONIST R	83752
L-ACTING-DRUG INCREASED		VASCULATURE SENSITIVITY RENIN	69192
ENAL FAILURE AND PATCHY		VASOCONSTRICTION CT AND MR FIN	35933
LOW/ NEURALLY MEDIATED		VASOCONSTRICTION DURING ISOME	137045
LUCOSE/ SPLANCHNIC AND		VASOCONSTRICTION DURING NEURO	108518
SSANT-DRUG SIDE EFFECTS		VASOCONSTRICTION PHARMACODYN	72010
PTOR ALPHA-1-B RECEPTOR		VASOCONSTRICTION RENAL RESISTA	96872
ADENOSINE A-2 RECEPTOR		VASOCONSTRICTION RENAL VASODIL	120229
RUG AUTOIMMUNE DISEASE		VASOCONSTRICTION T-CELL ACTIVA	59358
N RATE RENAL BLOOD FLOW		VASOCONSTRICTION/ A ROLE FOR E	59837
YNAMICS NEPHROTOXICITY		VASOCONSTRICTION/ IN-VIVO AND	97029
ENAL IMPAIRMENT HUMAN		VASOCONSTRICTION/ PLASMA ENDO	139757
LOOXYGENASE HUMAN RAM		VASOCONSTRICTOR ACTIVITY/ REGI	118397
MEDIA PHARMACOTOXICITY		VASOCONSTRICTOR INTRACELLULAR	23260
SFUNCTION HYPERTENSION		VASODILATATION RELAXATION RESP	85212
YNTHESIS RESOLUTION AND		VASODILATION ACTIVITY OF NOVEL	68430
RENAL VASOCONSTRICTION		VASODILATION GLOMERULAR FILTRA	120229
GMP OUTPUT NITRIC OXIDE		VASODILATION HYPERRESPONSIVENE	13701
ENZYME INHIBITOR-DRUG		VASODILATION HYPOTENSION/ PHAR	137725
EMATOCRIT/ EVIDENCE FOR		VASODILATION IN PRE-DIALYSIS P	94920
METABOLITES RAT RABBIT		VASODILATOR RESPONSE RENAL TUB	72218
S IN A RETROAORTIC LEFT		VEIN AND INCIDENTAL RIGHT CIRC	101782
CAL RESECTION PLANNING/		VEIN AND INFERIOR VENA CAVA TU	125120
THE TRANSITION BETWEEN		VEIN AND SUPRARENAL VEIN IN MA	74173
NCE IMAGING CASE REPORT		VEIN ANOMALIES RENAL CELL CARC	101782
CAVA INTERRUPTION WITH		VEIN COLLAR CONTINUATION CT AN	49409
AL LIGATION OF THE LEFT		VEIN IN THE DOG AN INAPPROPRIA	13593
HUMAN TUMOR DIAMETER		VEIN METASTASES SURVIVAL/ INFL	136258
TUBULAR REABSORPTION/		VEIN OXYGEN SATURATION IN RENA	108519
ISORDER/ PERIPHERAL AND		VEIN RENIN ACTIVITY IN PATIENT	73750
E EFFECT OF CAFFEINE ON		VEIN RENIN CONCENTRATION IN PA	49297
ORTAL VEIN HEPATIC VEIN		VEIN SUPERIOR MESENTERIC VEIN/	49366
UTE GLOMERULONEPHRITIS		VEIN THROMBOSIS ACUTE URATE NE	118335
PHY IN THE DIAGNOSIS OF		VEIN THROMBOSIS HUMAN GLOMER	94832
IC METHOD/ RETROAORTIC		VEIN WITH TUMOR THROMBUS MR F	101781
SYSTEM IN THE BLOOD OF		VEINS IN VASORENAL ARTERIAL HY	131108
W HUMAN ENDOTOXINEMIA		VESSEL DAMAGE GLOMERULAR MESA	118315
EX EVALUATION OF NATIVE		VESSELS AND RENAL ALLOGRAFTS R	106798
CROSCOPY/ INJURY OF RAT		VESSELS FOLLOWING EXTRACORPORE	94854
IDNEY WATER EXCRETION/		WATER HANDLING EVALUATED BY LI	23769
NSUMPTION LIVER WEIGHT		WEIGHT/ INFLUENCE OF DEHYDROEP	133155
TION OF PROTEINURIA AND		XANTHINE OXIDASE ACTIVITY BY D	118256
DIETARY PHOSPHATE LOAD		1 ALPHA-HYDROXYLASE VITAMIN SY	72093
IN RATS VIA STIMULATING		1 HYDROXYLASE ACTIVITY PARATHY	35997
LISA/ INHIBITION OF RAT		11-BETA HYDROXYSTEROID DEHYDRO	36044
N D HYDROXYLASES HUMAN		24 HYDROXYLASE TARGET CELL GEN	132877
M PHOSPHATE/ THE HUMAN		25 HYDROXYVITAMIN D-3-1-ALPHA-	140957
YTOLUENE ANTIDOTE-DRUG	**RENAL-ACTING**	AGENT ANTIURICEMIC PH	106263
ON ANTINEOPLASTIC AGENT		AGENT LUNG METASTASIS	113721
GENT IMMUNOLOGIC AGENT		AGENT NATURAL KILLER C	101934
OSPHATE WR-2721 RABBIT		AGENT PHARMACODYNAMI	72155
AN ANTINEOPLASTIC AGENT		AGENT TOXICITY PROFILE	79427
NDROGEN HORMONE AGENT		AGENT 5-ALPHA REDUCTAS	103702
ER CANCER REVIEW HUMAN		PHARMACOTHERAPY ANTI	102102
EAST CANCER COMPARISON		PHARMACOTHERAPY ANTI	102103
ER CANCER REVIEW HUMAN		PHARMACOTHERAPY ANTI	102104
NIDINE AND ANALOGS DOG		SODIUM REABSORPTION B	138373
HROTIC SYNDROME HUMAN	**RENAL-ACTING-DRUG**	/CLINICAL AND PA	9224
ND INCONTINENCE HUMAN		/CLINICAL STUDIE	92437
MMUNOSUPPRESSANT-DRUG		/EFFECT OF 15 DE	115809
NORMAL SUBJECTS HUMAN		/EFFECTS OF DOP	69189
TLET OBSTRUCTION HUMAN		/EFFECTS OF PINA	21262
UTY NEPHROPATHY HUMAN		/EFFICACY OF THE	33217
INAMIDE BENZBROMARONE		/EVALUATION OF	1860
HRITIS HUMAN FENOTEROL		/PARTUSISTEN IS	140862
CY VIRUS ANTIVIRAL-DRUG		ACQUIRED IMMUN	38055
S ENZYME INHIBITOR-DRUG		ALBUMIN NEPHRO	21258
L ENZYME INHIBITOR-DRUG		ANGIOTENSIN CON	9213
E ANTIHYPERTENSIVE-DRUG		ANTIATHEROGENI	103141

thesaurus, which means that IM uses a controlled vocabulary. This subject index in BA is called a KWIC (Key Word in Context) index. A type of natural language index, KWIC uses the language of the author. There are pros and cons for both of these types of indexes, and we will consider these next.

CONTROLLED VOCABULARY VERSUS NATURAL LANGUAGE (FREE TEXT) INDEXES

Strengths and weaknesses of searching for information in a controlled vocabulary index (e.g., IM) and a natural language index (e.g., the subject index of BA) are discussed below.

1. *Synonym control.* Consider the example ''renal stones.'' For IM, MeSH uses the term ''Kidney Calculi.'' In BA, the KWIC subject index is formed by taking the words from the title. The author's words are used. Where you discover the information depends on how the author described the topic. Because there are no binding rules that authors follow in writing their titles, you must look in several places for this topic: renal calculi, renal stones, kidney calculi, and kidney stones, as well as the singular. There are other possibilities. The author's title might have been ''Oxylates in the Urinary Tract'' and have no mention of renal or kidney. A significant burden is put upon searchers in a natural language index if they are looking for a fairly comprehensive coverage of his topic. If the searchers need only a sampling of articles, though, the natural language search may be faster and easier. The first step is eliminated. They do not need to check a controlled vocabulary (e.g., MeSH) before entering the subject index. It is not surprising to conclude that the answer to the question of which system of indexing is preferred depends on the information need of the patron.

2. *Singular and plural.* The same type of problem occurs here as it did with the synonyms. The author may use either the singular or the plural form of words. The example from BA above showed entries at ''renal stone'' as well as ''renal stones.'' In addition, other suffixes may be attached to words (e.g., *-ing*, *-ed*, *-ence*, *-ent*, *-tion*). Making matters more difficult are singulars and plurals like ''mouse'' and ''mice.'' These are widely separated in a large index like BA. When the words in a print index are not widely separated, the searcher probably has little difficulty. However, the situation changes for computer searching. The computer matches up the words entered letter by letter. Quite a lot of relevant information likely will not be seen. There are some remedies, however. Most computer systems allow for truncation. The searcher puts in the stem and gets the word with all the variant endings. Because not all plurals are signaled by *-s* and *-es*, other devices may be in order. Ovid Technologies (formerly BRS, Bibliographic Retrieval Services) offers a search option that lets you retrieve the singular and plural automatically. Setting ''Plurals-On'' at the start of a search will do this.

3. *Different spellings.* Several medical terms are spelled differently in British English and American English. ''Oesophagus'' and ''esophagus'' are very sim-

ilar spellings for the same part of the digestive system. Searchers would not be picking up everything in a free text index if they checked only the American spelling. This is a problem for both the computer users and the print users. In the alphabet, *o* is a long way from *e*. MEDLINE on Ovid features a solution to that problem, too. Setting ''Medspell-On'' picks up the British English and the American English. Remember, for both the singular-plural problem and the variable spellings, the controlled vocabulary brings all the variants together at one term.

4. *Hierarchical relationships.* Controlled vocabulary indexes offer advantages here. The searcher is looking for information about the leg. Knowing that the author may use a singular or plural, you search for ''leg'' or ''legs.'' However, it may very well be that the parts of the leg are your real interest. ''Thigh,'' ''knee,'' ''shin,'' and ''calf'' could be words in the title that you missed. A benefit of the controlled vocabulary is that a thesaurus displays the broader and narrower as well as the related terms. Your intent may have been to look for the leg as a whole, but it is just as likely you wanted information on the parts of the leg, too. In the indexing of documents by controlled vocabulary, remember the rule of specificity: If the article is just on the leg as a whole, it is indexed with ''Leg.'' If the article is on the knee, it is indexed under ''Knee'' and not also under ''Leg.'' From these comments, it seems you are bound to lose information with any index you use. There are two ways out of this. Do consult the thesaurus and search with the broader and narrower terms if you want to retrieve on both levels. Alternatively, when computer searching MEDLINE, use an Explode command (see Chapter 3) on the broad term to pick up both the broader term and the narrower terms.

5. *Specificity.* So far it seems not a lot can be said for natural language searching. Yet there are real advantages. This section looks at specificity somewhat differently than above. Controlled vocabularies may have a large number of terms. MeSH has over 17,000. Often, the searcher is looking for a topic that is even more specific than allowed for by large controlled vocabularies. The searcher wants articles on dachshunds, and the vocabulary offers only dogs. If limited to that vocabulary, you would need to look through all the ''dogs'' articles to find the few ''dachshunds'' ones. In the free text index, you could use any term that came into your head and probably retrieve something. There are hundreds of thousands of articles in the database, and some authors are likely to have used in their titles the words that you have chosen.

6. *Up-to-date vocabulary.* The controlled vocabulary will never be as up to date as the author's words. ''Wrongful Life'' appeared in several article titles over a three- or four-year period before it was made a MeSH term. New terms are immediately available for searching in the natural language indexes. Remember also that MeSH is unusual in that a new edition is published each year. Most other abstracting and indexing services put out thesauruses less frequently.

7. *Ease.* Natural language is simple. Just look in the index or type into the computer the word that comes to mind. There is not the same need to hunt for

the term chosen for the thesaurus. Nor do you need to make your topic fit the selection of terms offered by the controlled vocabulary. This needs to be clarified. Natural language is easier to use than controlled vocabulary if the need is for a few articles. Natural language is very hard if the need is for comprehensiveness.

8. *Lower cost to produce the index.* Natural language may be not only simpler to use but also quicker and cheaper for the index producer to develop. There is no need to employ well-trained and therefore relatively expensive indexers to examine and comprehend the material and then follow a set of exacting rules in applying the indexing vocabulary, as in the controlled language index. Just type the terms from the citations right into the computer and let the program store all the nontrivial words. This is close to what happens with the subject index of BA.

9. *Compound terms.* Compound terms may be used to aid in the retrieval of frequently requested topics. They are also helpful in eliminating faulty ''hits'' in the postcoordination of computer searching. With an uncontrolled vocabulary, a searcher may have to enter the terms ''library'' and ''school'' in the search. The retrieval consists of articles on ''library school'' and ''school library'' as well as other articles that happen to have both words in the record. A controlled vocabulary takes care of this problem fairly easily.

10. *Eliminate the divergent decisions of indexers, i.e. inconsistency.* The *MEDLARS Indexing Manual* has many guidelines for indexing. Indexing is difficult, but the access it provides is indispensable. There are not many opportunities to evaluate the indexing adequately. However, Funk and Reid (1983) found some interesting information concerning the indexing consistency for articles in MEDLINE. For various reasons, a group of 760 articles had been indexed two times. Funk and Reid compared the terms assigned to the same articles. They found differences in assigned terms. ''The highest consistency was 74.7%, for checktags, . . . the next highest category, central concept main headings at 61.1%. The lowest consistency was 33.8%, for main heading/subheading combinations'' (Funk and Reid 1983, 179). They conclude with this: ''It seems that, realistically, the upper level of consistency for any type of intellectual choice falls far below 100%. We believe that MEDLINE, with its excellent controlled vocabulary, exemplary quality control, and cadre of highly trained indexers, probably represents the state of the art in manually indexed data bases'' (Funk and Reid 1983, 183). The lesson is clear: Even with MEDLINE's superb system and controlled vocabulary, searchers must remember the inconsistency and tailor their searching appropriately. Despite problems with natural language searching, in contrast, searchers are not exposed to the varying interpretations of indexers.

SCIENCE CITATION INDEX

Recall that BA's KWIC index uses free text. Other types of indexes use free text also. *Dissertation Abstracts* has used a Key Word Out of Context (KWOC) index. This index, like KWIC, takes words from authors' titles, but it displays the words on the page a bit differently. The SCI calls its free text index ''Permuterm'' for its practice of permuting the words. Like BA's index, Permuterm selects words in the title as entry points. Permuterm offers the terms in pairs, unlike KWIC's positioning in a phrase of the title. Here is the entry in the Permuterm subject index of the 1991 SCI for articles about renal stones:

RENAL

STIMULATORY	Kimura K
STONE	Chang CP
	Fuss M
	Hess B
	Holm J
	Jabbour N
	Kiss D
	Thibert R
	Trinchie.A
	Urivetzk.M
	Wilson DM
STONE-FORM.	Simon D
STONES	Durlach R
	Ellis JH
	Karlsen SJ
	Kimmesmi.C
	Lee SK

Each nontrivial word is paired with every other nontrivial word of the title. One could consider this pairing of words print postcoordination because each search involves combining two terms. The word ''Renal,'' in our example, takes up about 80 columns in this index, without including the hyphenated entries. The small portion displayed above with ''Stone'' and ''Stone-Form.'' and ''Stones'' shows that there is not a great deal of vocabulary control here. The next step is to take the author's name at the right in the column and go the the source index of SCI for the full citation to the article in question. Note, too, when you arrive there, that the hyphenation is still ignored and the entry is at ''Kimmesmith C.'' If you go back to the Permuterm index and look at other combinations with ''renal,'' you will find an entry for ''Kimmesmi.C'' at ''detection,'' ''real-time,'' and ''sonography.'' ''Transducers'' and ''scanning'' were not included, perhaps because they were in the subtitle. This is again reminiscent of BA with its multitude of entry points. These other headings (e.g., ''sonography'') are main entry points in the alphabetical listing of the Permuterm index as well as being under "renal."

CITATION INDEXING

The somewhat traditional subject index of SCI is the Permuterm index. The citation index of SCI gives a totally different means of accessing the literature of the field. The ethic of science is the basis of the citation index. Investigations and experiments typically build incrementally on research done before. A small piece of information is added with each investigation, with each article. Authors are expected to acknowledge prior research. They must cite earlier works and then list the references at the end of their papers. Although no explicit instructions guide authors on the selection of their references, authors are expected to cite papers related to their own work. By looking at the works cited, the reader may get additional information about the subject.

The citation index enables the user to start with a cited reference instead of the citing paper. Take, for example, an article that may be of interest to us: Edward J. Huth, "Irresponsible Authorship and Wasteful Publication," *Annals of Internal Medicine* 104:257–259, 1986. Since we found this article of interest, articles that have cited this 1986 Huth paper may be of interest to us also. There is no law that an article once written will be cited. It may not even ever be read. So, we don't know if it will be cited in 1987 or 1992 or 1997 or 2002. Here is a part of a page where Huth EJ appears in the SCI citation index of 1992.

Huth EJ
59 J Clin Invest 38 1149

Mujais SK	Am J Physiol	262	F972	92

79 Ann Intern Med 90 120

Fletcher SW	J Intern M	232	223	92

(skipping a few entries)
86 Ann Intern Med 104 257

Freyschm.J	Radiologe	32	400	92
Halperin EC	Acad Med	67	850	92
Huth EJ	Diabet Care	15	1062	92
Kaplan P	Am J Phys M	71	81	92

(and more entries follow)

Huth EJ is found in alphabetical order. The two-digit numbers on the left of the rows represent the years of publication of the Huth papers and the listing is in chronological order. Go to the row "86 Ann Intern Med 104 257." This is the *Annals of Internal Medicine* article that we are looking for. Underneath that are several rows of names in alphabetical order. These are authors of more current papers (1992) that cited the 1986 paper by Huth. For example, Frcyschim.J wrote an article in *Radiologe* volume 32, page 400, 1992, that cited the Huth article. No first or middle names are used. The compilers of SCI just take the citing author's references and make little attempt to correct faulty citations in a paper. Not all of Huth's previous papers need to be indexed. They are included in SCI only if they were cited in 1992 by a journal that SCI indexes. To clarify, the journal of the cited paper does not need to be indexed by SCI. The *Science Citation Index* uses as entries all the citations it encounters in the citing papers—those source papers. Go to the source index of SCI to see the fuller citation.

Freyschmidt J
(GE) Paraethical and Nonethical Publication
Practices in Medicine
Radiologe 32(8):400–406 92 19R

This article happens to be in German. The "19R" refers to the number of references Freyschmidt's article has to other articles—one of which is the Huth article.

The citation index is not really an author index. It may be considered a type of subject index. The user finds articles on the subject in a different way. In addition, and important to the searcher, the whole area of language and vocabulary control is avoided. The user does not have to consult a controlled list of terms to make his subject terminology fit into the abstracting and indexing service's list of words. Also, the user does not have to try to guess what words an author might be using in the title of an article. This is a significant attribute that contributes to making this index well used by scientists. The SCI is expensive whether in paper, online, or CD-ROM format. The price notwithstanding, the scientists use it.

Another aspect of the citation index takes us back to Chapter 1, where we considered the scientist's need to publish in prestigious journals. We saw how publication in preferred journals is very important to a scientist's reputation, standing, and career. Yet much of the literature is not used. The citation index gives evidence of a contribution. That others cite your article demonstrates the utility of your work. Of course, we assume that the citing paper viewed your ideas positively. That need not be the case. Perhaps the authors citing your article believed your work to be full of errors and pointed that out. Such negative citations are the minority, however. Scientists whose works are cited often are pleased and gratified, and they happily point out the citations at promotion time. Scientists will also cite their own earlier papers because they build on what they did before. Not surprisingly, citing oneself does not have the same impact as being cited by someone else.

BEYOND IM, BA, AND SCI

Index Medicus and *Biological Abstracts* are the two primary abstracting and indexing services for biomedicine in North America. The *Science Citation Index* provides a unique and useful orientation. Other major indexes in biomedicine and related disciplines are covered next. Be familiar with them. For purposes of comparison, the same categories are presented for each: producer, subject scope, publication types and coverage, approximate cost and frequency, computer counterpart, and comments about use and indexing.

—*Biological Abstracts/RRM (Reports, Reviews, Meetings)* (BA/RRM)
Producer: BIOSIS.
Subject Scope: same as *Biological Abstracts.*
Publication Types and Coverage: journal review articles; technical reports; government documents; abstracts and papers from symposia; bibliographies; book chapters. Together with BA, BA/RRM indexes over 500,000 citations annually from over 6,000 serials.
Cost and Frequency: about $3,000; semimonthly.
Computer Counterpart: included in BIOSIS Database.
Comments: BA/RRM indexes the meetings abstracts as well as the full papers published from meetings. It is useful as a way to get at nonjournal material in biomedicine. Same indexing as BA. Does not have abstracts.

—*Hospital and Health Administration Index*
Former title (through 1994): *Hospital Literature Index.*
Producer: American Hospital Association with the National Library of Medicine.
Subject Scope: administrative, legal, organizational, and financial aspects of health care.
Publication Types and Coverage: English-language journal articles. Separate section for books, audiovisuals, and theses.
Cost and Frequency: $300; three issues per year.
Computer Counterpart: Health Planning and Administration.
Comments: nice complement to IM for issues such as the delivery, financing, and insuring of health care. In other words, useful for the ongoing health care debate and controversy. Indexed with MeSH.

—*International Nursing Index* (INI)
Producer: American Journal of Nursing Company. Sponsored by the American Nurses' Association. Published in cooperation with the National Library of Medicine.
Subject Scope: nursing.
Publication Types and Coverage: over 270 nursing journals plus articles from other journals in IM and *Hospital and Health Administration Index.* International and does include foreign-language articles. Also has lists of books and dissertations.
Cost and Frequency: $250; quarterly.
Computer Counterpart: included in MEDLINE.
Comments: MeSH is used for indexing INI. Annual cumulation contains a "Nursing Thesaurus." This consists of "see" and "see also" headings that link common nursing terms to MeSH headings. From 1986 through 1990, INI contained the *Nursing Citation Index* (from ISI). INI is known as the "Green Index." Note: nurses are the largest group of health care professionals.

—*Index to Dental Literature* (IDL)
Producer: American Dental Association with the National Library of Medicine.

Subject Scope: dentistry.

Publication Types and Coverage: about 20,000 journal articles indexed in 1992: 12,000 from dental journals and 8,000 from nondental journals. Also has lists of books and dissertations.

Cost and Frequency: $200; quarterly.

Computer Counterpart: included in MEDLINE.

Comments: MeSH used for indexing and layout looks the same as IM.

—*Cumulative Index to Nursing and Allied Health Literature* (CINAHL)

Producer: CINAHL Information Systems, Glendale, CA.

Subject Scope: as the title indicates, includes nursing and more, e.g., medical and laboratory technology, health education, medical records, occupational therapy, and rehabilitation.

Publication Types and Coverage: over 500 journals plus books, dissertations, and conference proceedings. Includes publications of the American Nurses' Association and the National League for Nursing. New format in 1993 has all the different types of citations in one section. Before that there were separate lists for books, journal articles, and so on.

Cost and Frequency: $260; bimonthly.

Computer Counterpart: CINAHL.

Comments: has own thesaurus, but is hierarchical like MeSH. Has alphabetical entries, trees, and permuted sections (Brenner and McKinin 1989). This is the "Red Index." Note: One of the subjects it covers is health sciences librarianship. Includes *Bulletin of the Medical Library Association*, *Health Libraries Review*, *Medical Reference Services Quarterly*, *Library Journal*, and *Serials Librarian*.

—*Chemical Abstracts* (CA)

Producer: Chemical Abstracts Service.

Subject Scope: chemistry, but stretches its coverage into biology and medicine (e.g., drugs).

Publication Types and Coverage: journal articles, symposia publications, books, audiovisuals, technical reports, patents. The biggest abstracting and indexing service covering over 15,000 sources.

Cost and Frequency: over $16,000; weekly.

Computer Counterpart: CAS Online and other designations.

Comments: *Index Guide* is the publication used for vocabulary control. Many access points in CA: molecular formula, CAS registry number (on computer), patent number, as well as substance index, subject index, and author index. *Chemical Abstracts Service Source Index* (CASSI) is very helpful for abbreviations and libraries' holdings.

—*Excerpta Medica* (EM)

Producer: Excerpta Medica of Elsevier Science Publishers.

Subject Scope: biomedicine.

Publication Types and Coverage: journals. 3,500 journals.

Cost and Frequency: $27,600. Comes in 41 abstract journals that can be purchased separately (e.g., *Gastroenterology*, *Cancer*, and *Surgery*).

Computer Counterpart: EMBASE.

Comments: international coverage like IM but provides greater coverage for European journals. Very good for drug literature. Years ago EM was thought to be much less current than IM. That disparity is not so great now.

—*Current Contents* (CC)

Producer: Institute for Scientific Information.

Subject Scope: two of the titles for CC: *Current Contents: Clinical Medicine* and *Current Contents: Life Sciences*.

Publication Types and Coverage: tables of contents of journals and a few books. Clinical Medicine, 900 journals; Life Sciences, 1,250 journals.

Cost and Frequency: $500 per CC title; weekly.

Computer Counterpart: available on diskette as well as online. There are, in fact, several journal contents alerting services now available on computer. The computerized services through Internet access have a competitive advantage over the paper product.

Comments: CC is an alerting service as opposed to a traditional abstracting and indexing service. Reproduces tables of contents of journals. For paper tools, this usually has the shortest lag time.

—*Psychological Abstracts* (PA)

Producer: American Psychological Association.

Subject Scope: psychology.

Publication Types and Coverage: journal articles, books, and book chapters. 1,300 journals.

Cost and Frequency: $1,375; monthly.

Computer Counterpart: PsycINFO.

Comments: endorses itself for a variety of medical subjects: "behavioral causes, effects, or treatment of disease; doctor-patient interaction; drug and alcohol abuse and rehabilitation; drug therapy; mental health; professional health personnel issues; psychiatry; psychopharmacology" (American Psychological Association 1992, sect. 1, p. 4). Also useful for nursing and allied health issues.

—*International Pharmaceutical Abstracts* (IPA)

Producer: American Society of Hospital Pharmacists.

Subject Scope: pharmaceutical information.

Publication Types and Coverage: about 800 journals.

Cost and Frequency: $425; semimonthly.

Computer Counterpart: International Pharmaceutical Abstracts.

Comments: directed to the pharmacist; also an additional source of drug information for a wider audience.

—*Cambridge Scientific Abstracts*

Producer: Cambridge Information Group.

Subject Scope: biomedicine and beyond.

Publication Types and Coverage: journal articles and conference papers.

Cost and Frequency: sources covering biology and medicine, over $15,000 if received all.

Computer Counterpart: CSA Life Sciences Collection and others.

Comments: similar to EM. Has many abstract journals that can be subscribed to separately (e.g., *Immunology Abstracts*, *Virology and AIDS Abstracts*, and *BioEngineering Abstracts*).

PROBLEMS OF TIMELINESS

MeSH is updated every year. In 1963 there were 5,700 terms, whereas now there are over 17,000. The annual renovation of the vocabulary is an impressive accomplishment. It is your responsibility to keep up to date on these changes. Also, some rules of indexing change over time. Keeping current on the vocabulary and indexing rules is necessary. What about the vocabulary and rules of five years ago? of fifteen years ago? Your print IM of five years ago was not recalled by the manufacturer to be brought into compliance with the new rules and new terminology. Earlier material on MEDLINE may be retrieved with the old indexing rules and vocabulary. You not only need to know current rules and to be prepared to learn future rules but also to be familiar with past practices. The annotated alphabetic section of MeSH, designed for computerized searching, will provide some assistance.

MEDICAL TERMINOLOGY: INDEXER AND SEARCHER

How are MeSH terms chosen? The National Library of Medicine uses print sources and experts in the various fields as authorities. *Dorland's Illustrated Medical Dictionary*, a general medical dictionary, is another source. You should familiarize yourself with the major medical dictionaries (Putney and Roper 1994). A list of the print authorities can be found in the introduction of each edition of MeSH. The subject headings in MeSH are chosen to aid retrieval of articles for users of print and computer products. Beyond understanding how the controlled vocabulary terms are selected, it would also be good to know what terms physicians actually use in their medical practices. What is their terminology when communicating with each other? with their patients? What terminology is used in the patient's medical record? There is a logic to the formation of medical terms. For instance, words are often constructed from Greek and Latin roots, prefixes, and suffixes. Medical librarians should familiarize themselves with the terminology used by physicians. One way to do this is to use a book on medical terminology, and there are programmed texts available for this purpose (Smith and David 1991).

Earlier it was noted that at NLM an indexer previously could make a check on a form to select the check tags such as HUMAN or CHILD or CASE REPORT. This served to remind indexers about some frequently used concepts. For the rest of the subjects, the indexer consulted MeSH books and applied the rules learned. The indexing now is done on a computer screen. Putting this procedure in a program instead of on a piece of paper adds another dimension to indexing. "If the indexer adds the MeSH heading 'DOG DISEASES' to an article, the program will automatically add the check tags 'DOGS' and 'ANIMAL.' . . . Various warnings, reminders, and suggestions may be invoked by the program whenever specific headings or qualifiers are assigned" (National Library of Medicine 1993c). The MedIndEx (Medical Indexing Expert) Project at the National Library of Medicine is the name given to this initiative. Automatic indexing has been something librarians and information scientists have been looking into for several years. MedIndEx is designed to give the human indexer a ''smart'' helper. The rules of indexing are embedded in the program for the human indexer to use (Humphrey 1989).

The other side of the story is on the searching end. Knowing the terminology that health professionals use enables us to serve them better. We need to recognize that physicians and other practitioners talk and write in free text, not with controlled vocabulary. We need to enable them to retrieve information easily. It has been important for us to learn the controlled vocabulary of MeSH. We have discussed at length the variations in retrieval for controlled vocabulary and free text indexes. Will health professionals use the controlled vocabularies in their searches? We assume they will not. So how can we help them in their information retrieval? At this time, NLM is using the Unified Medical Language System (UMLS) in an attempt to address this problem. The first step in the UMLS project is to determine the varied terminologies used by the health professional community to describe the same things. After this medical thesaurus is organized, investigations will be made to see how this information can be implemented in the computer systems. NLM plans to integrate this UMLS information in searching systems in 1996. The next chapter considers computer searching of the literature by us and also by our patrons.

On the Internet, many discussion groups have been set up centered around specific interests. One useful group is INDEX-L, where indexers, librarians, and others discuss a variety of topics in indexing. Here you can check on what is being talked about concerning automatic indexing, medical indexing, or even MedIndEx.

THE HISTORICAL PERSPECTIVE: FROM ORGANIZING AND INDEXING TO COMPUTERIZATION

For a long time, as we know, the focus of our field has been on identifying and obtaining journal articles. Now, medical librarians and our patrons are on the verge of being able to effectively enter plain English requests into the computer and retrieve full-text information at their desktop. Medical libraries have been leaders in implementing computer searching and telecommunications. It is useful, perhaps necessary, and even interesting to know how we got to this point. A history of the evolution of medical librarianship is related here through the growth and the development of one library and its services and the leadership and vision of a handful of individuals.

Few medical libraries existed in the early 1800s. Physicians typically referred to their own collections. The U.S. Army surgeon general, Joseph Lovell, did that, too. Part of his job was to provide books and journals to the physicians stationed at military posts around the country. He died in 1836, and the small collection of medical books and journals in his office was used by his successor. By the end of the Civil War, the collection had grown modestly to around 2,000 volumes, which included about 50 journals. At this time a young physician,

John Shaw Billings, took over the running of that little library. His legacy is a great national library, NLM, and the premier tool for the organization of the medical literature, the IM.

At first Billings was just one among a number of physicians who would order materials for the library. After Billings had been at his post a few years, Surgeon General Joseph K. Barnes asked Billings to take, as one of his duties, the responsibility for the library. Barnes did not seem to give Billings any grand mandate. However, shortly thereafter Billings decided on this course: ''I wish in time to make the Library of this office as complete as possible'' (Miles 1982, 29). He meant it. Billings began a campaign to acquire all the medical books, pamphlets, and journals he could find. He wrote letters to physicians all over the country. Did they have medical literature to donate to the library, he asked. Were they thinking of retirement and would they send their collections to him in Washington, D.C., he also asked. He sent his assistants on scavenger hunts. They approached retired physicians and widows of physicians. They looked in people's attics hunting for materials to send back to Billings's library. The collection grew: to 14,000 in 1871; to 25,000 in 1873; and to 51,000 in 1880 (Miles 1982, 177). Funds available for this purpose were minimal, and the collection was acquired for amazingly small outlays of money.

Billings was not solely involved with collection development and acquisitions. He shared the vital concern medical librarians have had through succeeding generations: How can we help get the information into the physicians' hands when they need it? Not irrelevantly, he had encountered this difficulty in finding information when he was in school preparing his dissertation. He now set about indexing the medical literature—books, pamphlets, and journal articles. His associate, Fielding Garrison, described Billings' activities thus:

> Almost every day, a government van would leave a wagon load of bound periodicals at his residence in Georgetown and the next morning would find their principal articles, cases, and essays carefully checked, by lead-pencil markings, for the copyists in the office. This night work continued until the gigantic task of indexing all the bound periodicals was accomplished, but even in the later days, when he had only the current unbound periodicals to deal with, Billings still continued to take some of these home in his overcoat pocket, or to have them sent up in baskets, for checking. (Miles 1982, 112–113)

Even Billings could not do everything. One person could not index the whole collection. He solicited help from physicians all over the country and had them participate in this indexing project. He was also very willing to impart to them the guidelines for indexing that he wanted used. From his collecting and indexing, Billings started two monumental publications: *Index-Catalogue of the Library of the Surgeon General's Office* and *Index Medicus*.

INDEX-CATALOGUE OF THE LIBRARY OF THE SURGEON GENERAL'S OFFICE

Billings had the idea of creating a catalog of all the holdings in the library—the books, the pamphlets, and even the articles contained within the journal issues. With a print catalog, copies could be supplied to physicians throughout the country. The doctors could look in the catalog and find the publications on any specific topic they needed information on. Then, after identifying the item, the doctor could write to this newly created "National Medical Library." Billings would then send out the requested materials. It was a terrific idea and a huge undertaking—and it would cost a lot of money. Although Billings may have looked on the library as his own, it was still a government facility. Funds were not easily obtained. To create his great library, Billings had relied mostly on donations, exchanges, and small expenditures.

Billings decided he needed to garner support for his project. He had a plan, and he began the campaign. He compiled the *Specimen Fasciculus of a Catalogue of the National Medical Library.* This was a sample for the complete catalog he wanted to produce. It contained index entries to some of those articles, books, and pamphlets. He had a number of copies printed and sent out. Billings was careful to send them to people who might be able to exert some influence on Congress. He needed to obtain a good-sized appropriation to produce his catalog. It worked. The physicians saw in the project the immense resource it would be. This would be a way for them to identify the sources for answers that they needed in their practice of medicine, and it also provided a way to get the books, journals, and pamphlets. This is the same need we have today, and we are still working to improve the process.

With initial enthusiasm great, the funds came. But the funding through the years was not always overwhelming. The project was long and took many years. The first volume of the *Index-Catalogue of the Library of the Surgeon General's Office* was published in 1880 and contained A-Berlinski. The alphabet was completed, and the first series finished in 1895 with volume 16, W-Zythus. It "contained 174,364 author and 168,557 subject entries for books and pamphlets. It also contained subject entries for 511,112 journal articles. The library collection at this time consisted of 116,847 books and 191,598 pamphlets" (Waserman 1972, 552). The second series was begun and took from 1896 to 1916. The production of the third series continued from 1918 to 1932. Then there came a fourth series and a fifth series. After that, the project was halted. The *Index-Catalogue*, it should be emphasized, indexed not only the library's books but also its pamphlets and journal articles. Today we do have a cumulated record of the holdings of the library's books. It is updated weekly and can be searched from computers all over the country. This database, called CATLINE, is an important part of the NLM system and we will talk more about it. In contrast to the frequent updating of computerized databases possible today, the beginning of the twentieth century witnessed the development of a catalog that took fifteen to twenty years to complete the sequence of the alphabet from A to Z.

THE HISTORY OF IM AND RELATED MEDICAL INDEXES

Billings could see that the *Index-Catalogue* was going to take many years to produce. Meanwhile, physicians still needed to learn about new findings, case studies, and research to keep up-to-date. To supply information about the current year's literature, Billings and Robert Fletcher worked on another project. In 1879 *Index Medicus, a Monthly Classified Record of the Current Medical Literature of the World* was born. It covered 600 journals and 20,000 articles. The *Index-Catalogue* and IM had different arrangements. The *Index-Catalogue* interspersed authors and subjects in one alphabet. It was not searchable by the authors of journal articles. *Index Medicus*, which was set up for the journal literature, had a subject arrangement with an author index.

Although the importance of IM today cannot be overstated, from its inception and through much of its history, IM found funds difficult to come by. Unlike the *Index-Catalogue*, IM was not supported by government appropriations, and not enough individuals subscribed to make it a financially secure publication. In addition, in 1895 Billings left the National Medical Library, as he called it. *Index Medicus* ceased publication in 1899, but other organizations came forward to help produce it, and in 1903 it resumed with financial help from the Carnegie Institution. It did not hurt that at this time Billings was a trustee of the Carnegie Institution. With this new source of funds and Fielding Garrison joining Robert Fletcher as co-editor, IM came back to life. Librarians knew the importance of IM. The librarian of the New York Academy of Medicine wrote in the official publication of the newly formed Association of Medical Librarians (now known as the Medical Library Association), *Medical Library and Historical Journal*: "Since 1899, when the *Index Medicus* was discontinued, this task [keeping up-to-date] has been a difficult one. The importance of renewing this publication, now being undertaken by the Carnegie Institute, cannot be overestimated in its practical value to Medical Science" (Brownne 1903, 34).

In 1916, the American Medical Association (AMA) began a new publication, the *Quarterly Cumulative Index to Current Medical Literature*. It covered 150 journals and 10,000 journal articles. By 1925, it grew to 300 journals and 25,000 articles. At that time, IM covered around 45,000 journal articles. The *Quarterly Cumulative Index to Current Medical Literature* also benefited from the tireless resolve of dedicated individuals. Over a period of 40 years, three people were largely responsible for its production: Helen Hutchinson Green, Marjorie Hutchins Moore, and Magdalene Freydar Hodgson.

Organizations as well as publications were changing. In 1922, the Library of the Surgeon General's Office became the Army Medical Library. In 1927 IM merged with AMA's *Quarterly Cumulative Index to Current Medical Literature* to form the *Quarterly Cumulative Index Medicus* (QCIM). The AMA took over production in 1932. The QCIM was indexing 90,000 articles annually by 1939. The Friends of the Army Medical Library began a weekly publication, the *Current List of Medical Literature*, in 1941. Its purpose was to promote current awareness and had tables of contents of medical journals. In 1950, it became a monthly.

The Army Medical Library became the Armed Forces Medical Library in 1952. Changes in names and sponsors did not solve the problems that IM, under its various names, had. The QCIM lagged behind. In the 1950s, it belied its name and started to appear only twice a year. Even worse, it was three years behind in its indexing. Meanwhile, in 1950 the decision to stop the publication of the *Index-Catalogue* was made. The last volume, the sixty-first issued since 1880, appeared in 1961. The preface of that volume indicates the total number of publications included during those 80 years of publication (Rogers 1961, iii):

Books and Pamphlets	538,509
Journal Articles	2,556,036

NATIONAL LIBRARY OF MEDICINE (NLM)

NLM was moved physically and organizationally at various times over the years. Funds for the library and for the indexing operations were usually sparse. Buildings for the library were also a concern. For instance, in 1933 Dr. Harvey Cushing wrote to President Roosevelt:

> You of course know all about the Surgeon-General's Library, for which John S. Billings was originally responsible. It is the only great medical library in the world, and the *Index Medicus* and the *Index-Catalogue* are probably more widely used throughout the world than any other medical books which have ever been published since the book of Isaiah. (Dupree 1957, 347–348)

Cushing then went on to plead for a new building because the collections were in physical danger from substandard conditions.

Finally, in 1956, help for IM and the library arrived. Senators Lister Hill (AL) and John Kennedy (MA) sponsored a bill to create the National Library of Medicine. It was put under the Public Health Service. In 1968 NLM moved organizationally under the National Institutes of Health. The construction of a new building was authorized in the bill. The library moved into the new building in Bethesda, Maryland, in 1962. ''The National Library of Medicine (NLM) is the world's largest research library in a single scientific and professional field. The Library collects materials exhaustively in all major areas of the health sciences and to a lesser degree in such areas as chemistry, physics, botany and zoology'' (National Library of Medicine 1995a). The NLM statistics for the year ending September 30, 1994, are impressive: collection (book and nonbook), 5,016,000; serial titles received, 23,250; articles indexed for MEDLINE, 368,000; and computerized searches of all databases 6,890,000 (Mehnert 1995, 167). John Shaw Billings always intended his library to serve the nation and referred to it as the National Medical Library. The U.S. government finally put into law what Billings had put into practice ninety years earlier.

The solutions were at hand for the problems of the medical indexes. The QCIM and the *Current List of Medical Literature* stopped publication in 1960. *Index Medicus* resumed on a monthly basis at NLM. The AMA continued to publish the annual cumulation, *Cumulated Index Medicus*, for several more years. In 1965 NLM took over responsibility for that as well. In the 1950s and early 1960s came much debate on how to produce IM more efficiently. Still foremost was IM's original purpose—to get the information to physicians and researchers on a timely basis—and this was not being achieved. Exciting advances were at hand.

THE ROAD TO MEDLARS

Harold Jones headed NLM from 1936 to 1945. In 1943 he arranged for a study of the library to be done by outside librarians. The American Library Association (ALA) appointed a survey team of six librarians, who made several trips to the Library. The surveyors found many difficulties and issued many recommendations. Many practices were not in accordance with current library methods. Part of the problem stemmed from insufficient funding. They also saw the need for training in librarianship. This made sense to Joseph McNinch, the director from 1946 to 1949. He decided it would be best to have a person trained in both medicine and librarianship. Frank Bradway Rogers, a surgeon in the military at this time, applied for the position at the library. After his transfer to the library, he was sent to the Columbia University School of Library Service. In 1949 McNinch left and Rogers became the director.

Rogers involved himself in the indexing operation. The Welch Medical Indexing Project was set up at Johns Hopkins and supported by the Army Medical Library. At that time much investigation was going on in indexing theory and information retrieval. For instance, Mortimer Taube was one influential voice, and the Medical Library listened to his ideas on "uniterms" and "coordinate indexing." "Dr. Rogers set for himself an intellectual challenge which has occupied his professional career—to master the principles underlying the construction and use of formal systems of subject headings in the medical sciences" (Adams 1972, 528). In 1959 Rogers settled on MeSH for use in both the cataloging of books and the indexing of journal articles. The upgrading of the indexing vocabulary was one thing. Rogers was also interested in utilizing the computer, and he assigned his deputy director, Scott Adams, to the project. Adams worked with government contractors to investigate the possibilities. General Electric arranged with the Photon Company to develop a high-speed phototypesetter that used magnetic tape as the input. Named GRACE (Graphic Arts Composing Equipment), the phototypesetter was first used in the production of IM in August 1964. Perhaps visionaries could see the future of online searching. More practically, however, the main objective of utilizing this new process with computers was to produce IM more quickly and reliably. The computerized system was named MEDLARS (Medical Literature Analysis and Retrieval System).

BATCH SEARCHING AND BIBLIOGRAPHIES

A computerized database was accumulating. Hundreds of thousands of journal article citations from thousands of journals were being stored in MEDLARS. The huge software industry of today did not exist then. NLM contracted with the System Development Corporation (SDC) to devise ways to search the database. The first way to search was not the online, interactive method that we use today. It was a batch system. Queries were organized into terms meaningful to the system and fed into the computer in groups of searches. It took 40 minutes for the computer to go through all the tapes. Therefore, economically, it was wise to batch several searches to be fed in at the same time. A physician from anywhere in the country could request NLM to search on a specified topic. Specially trained search analysts would translate the query into combinations of headings. Turnaround time for these searches was about a month counting the mail in both directions. With the newfound ease of production, NLM also generated subsets of IM on topics like toxicology, rheumatology, and diabetes. These ongoing bibliographies were distributed in the same way as IM itself. This powerful tool was the forerunner of online searching that proudly came into librarianship in the 1970s.

AIM/TWX AND MEDLINE

The opportunity to order tailored bibliographies that would be prepared in a few weeks was a great service that NLM innovated. To make the service more timely, NLM toyed with the idea of locating MEDLARS centers in various parts of the country. In 1970 NLM came up with a different approach. For this project, several elements needed to be brought together. First, groups of medical librarians around the country had been trained in the searching vocabulary, so that they could assist patrons in the formulation of their searches. Second, and quite conveniently, many libraries of all types had been using a teletypewriter exchange machine (TWX) to transmit interlibrary loan requests among themselves. Third was the development of an appropriate database. NLM created a subset of IM, the *Abridged Index Medicus* (AIM). This contained the citations to articles from 100 English-language journals that represented the prime publications in clinical medicine. NLM took the trained personnel (the medical librarians around the country), the communications network (TWX), the database (AIM), and the searching software of MEDLARS (ELHILL, named for Senator Lister Hill) to create an online database searching system, AIM/TWX. It was an experiment that did not last very long, because AIM/TWX was an immediate success. Later in 1971 a fuller database was made available and MEDLINE was born. MEDLINE stands for MEDlars onLINE (MEDLINE will be examined in Chapter 3).

Another important step in the computerization of the medical literature took place at the State University of New York (SUNY). The SUNY Biomedical Communication Network became operational in 1968. Its system included the MEDLARS tapes from NLM. Libraries connected by dedicated lines were able to search the database from their remote locations. This was a beginning of online searching. The AIM/TWX experiment added the capability of using regular telephone lines, and that made the system available from any place in the country (Pizer 1984).

ADDENDUM

Skip to the present. Note that the information given a few pages ago on the size and activities of NLM is for 1993 and 1994. That is out of date. You can pull up current information quickly and conveniently with electronic fact sheets. Use your Internet connection to travel to NLM's Home Page or Gopher with the following:

http://www.nlm.nih.gov/factsheets.dir/factsheets.html
or
gopher://gopher.nlm.nih.gov/11/nlminfo/factsheets/

3

Computerized Bibliographic Searching: MEDLINE and Beyond

INTRODUCTION

Chapter 2 journeyed the traditional road through the paper indexes to the biomedical journal literature. As you look at the index tables in your library, you see that this year's monthly issues of IM and other indexes, too, are in remarkably good physical condition (assuming here that they have not yet been cancelled). Pages are not torn, the covers are still on, and all the issues are sitting just where they were yesterday and last week. Those volumes are not used as much as they used to be. Your patrons are searching MEDLINE and other computerized databases instead of using the paper indexes. The indexing practices and policies discussed in Chapter 2 for the paper indexes are still important as we move to the computer keyboard. We will see that shortly. Those paper abstracting and indexing tools are available by computer, and there are in fact dozens, if not hundreds, of secondary sources relevant to the biomedical sciences. Fewer and fewer indexes are still available only in paper. Other indexes are not available in paper at all; they can be accessed only via computer (e.g., *Mental Health Abstracts*).

The computer index and the paper index do not always contain identical information. Along with the more numerous access points, the computer file may contain more data. For example, we saw that MEDLINE includes within it the citations from the *International Nursing Index* and the *Index to Dental Literature* in addition to IM. Many of the records in MEDLINE contain abstracts, whereas IM does not have abstracts. Similarly, not all the citations in the database EMBASE are in its print publication, *Excerpta Medica*. This chapter focuses mainly on ways of searching MEDLINE and will help you become familiar with IM and MEDLINE. However, it is up to you to know what else is available because IM and MEDLINE do not have everything that your biomedical clientele need. You will want to consult manuals and attend training sessions to get the additional information you will need. Here, specific directions are presented that take the searcher from the vocabulary of the print index to the use of terms on the computer. Successful computer searches depend on mastering the system, knowing the database, and managing the interaction with the patron. One variable in this has to do with the nature of the patron's request. Often physicians will want a few ''good'' articles, so one of our goals is to find techniques to get just those good, pertinent articles. Other requestors will want to get everything you can find on a topic, and you will have the devices to search comprehensively. Which system or systems will you be using?

ACCESS TO MEDLINE

There are choices for computer access to most of the abstracting and indexing services. Today the two main avenues are online and CD-ROM. Online vendors for MEDLINE include but are not limited to NLM; DIALOG Information Services; Ovid Technologies, which took over Bibliographic Retrieval Services (BRS) in 1994; PaperChase (Beth Israel Hospital); LEXIS-NEXIS; and OCLC's EPIC and FirstSearch. Some of the CD-ROM vendors are SilverPlatter; Aries Systems; CDP, which in 1995 changed its name to Ovid Technologies for the parent company; DIALOG Information Services, whose parent became Knight Ridder; and EBSCO Electronic Information. The MEDLINE database on all the vendors is the database produced by NLM. In other words, MEDLINE contains the same bibliographic records whether it is mounted on the computer at NLM or DIALOG or any other vendor. Whereas the producer of an index usually kept the role of producer and distributor of the paper products, several vendors now offer access to the computerized databases. In Chapter 2, we saw the development of AIM/TWX and MEDLINE, which was initially made available directly from NLM and was also searchable via the SUNY system. For several years this was the only way to search the MEDLINE database. In the 1970s private companies began to act as vendors of databases. DIALOG Information Retrieval Service, SDC, and BRS were companies that arranged leases with numerous database producers. Libraries and other patrons obtained computer access to these databases online through those and other vendors. Over the years some databases were offered directly online by the producer (e.g., NLM) or by a vendor of several data bases (e.g., DIALOG) or by both the producer and the vendor.

The 1980s brought another important step in the dissemination of journal article information—the abstracting and indexing services on CD-ROMs. The compact disk presents a dense storage medium for bibliographic data. The laser technology to ''read'' the disks has brought this very convenient form of access into the library. The producers of the databases have entered into agreements with more vendors, such as SilverPlatter, to put their databases in CD-ROM form. Leasing arrangements made by libraries resemble annual journal subscriptions. Online has had both the advantage and disadvantage of charges based on use. This variability has either caused problems for libraries' budgets or scared many librarians from using online services. The CD-ROMs have brought back the fixed costs to which libraries had been accustomed. One other mode of access has become more economically and technologically feasible for individual institutions: Universities have begun to lease tapes from producers and put those databases on their own mainframe computers for the use of their staffs and students.

Although the same MEDLINE database is on all the systems, vendors add their own searching software and techniques for information retrieval. The system variations offer alternative advantages, and we will look at some of these searching variables. The database producer and system vendor supply information that you will need that is beyond the scope of this chapter. Use their documentation and training. Here, we will start with some basic and useful concepts. First, however, the ideas discussed in the last chapter about the MeSH vocabulary and indexing principles need to be expanded on for computer searching.

THE SEARCH PROCESS AND BOOLEAN LOGIC

The process of computer searching starts with a search request. Since the advent of online searching, most searches in biomedicine have been for bibliographies, that is, for tailored lists of journal article citations. This is not always the case and may become even less so in the future. Other requests may lead us to (1) full-text databases and (2) data databases (e.g., numbers, toxicity, molecular structures, protein sequences). Here is a sample request for the tailored bibliographic search: ''Is marijuana helpful in alleviating some side effects of cancer treatments?'' We need to put the question into a form that the computer can handle. (Later in the chapter, some ideas will be presented on natural language processing—searching with regular English sentences.) There has to be something about cancer in the article and something about marijuana in the same article for the journal article to be helpful to us. The search statement makes use of Boolean operators. The first Boolean operator is ''AND.'' ''AND'' makes the search more restrictive. For example:

100,000 articles on cancer
800 articles marijuana
combine cancer ''AND'' marijuana: 8 articles

There are only eight articles that include both cancer and marijuana. This demonstrates the power of postcoordination with computer manipulation. The searcher may put in as many ''AND's'' as desired. The total number of articles retrieved will keep going down with additional ''AND's.''

cancer ''AND'' marijuana ''AND'' female: 3 articles

To broaden the search, use another Boolean operator: ''OR.''

800 articles on marijuana
400 articles on marihuana [to account for different spellings]
1,000 articles on cannabis
marijuana ''OR'' marihuana ''OR'' cannabis: 1,300 articles

''OR'' means ''either or.'' In the example above, 800 plus 400 plus 1,000 did not equal 2,200. Some articles contained more than one of the three words. Each article would be counted only once no matter how many of the three words were in it. Often, ''OR's'' are used first in the gathering of sets in preparation for an ''AND'' to follow.

(1) marijuana or marihuana or cannabis	1,300
(2) cancer	100,000
(3) 1 and 2	10

To eliminate articles from a set of retrieval, use the Boolean operator ''NOT.'' The NLM's system calls it ''AND NOT.''

1,000 articles on cannabis
4,000 articles on cocaine
cannabis ''AND NOT'' cocaine: 800 articles

There are 800 articles that include cannabis and also had nothing about cocaine in them. Two hundred articles on cannabis were removed because they also discussed cocaine. A consumer warning usually comes with a system's version of ''NOT.'' ''NOT'' may do more than you wish, so it should be used judiciously. In this example, articles that happened to include cocaine may also have had pertinent information on cannabis. In other words, you may be getting rid of more information than you intended.

The power of computer searching has come from these simple Boolean operators. A problem of ''AND'' is that it specifies that only two words or ideas be included in the record of an article. The two must be present, but you are unable to direct a relationship between them. A searching system will often also include proximity operators to yield more refined retrieval. The proximity operators can specify that the terms be close together, or adjacent, in a record. To be able to show a more sophisticated relationship would often be very helpful. These operators are what we have to work with at this time.

Here are some steps in a simple Boolean search on MEDLINE (1991 through January 1994). The accompanying numbers represent the count of the journal articles with that concept.

1) KIDNEY CALCULI	779
2) LITHOTRIPSY	1098
3) 1 and 2	311
4) 3 and MALE	181
5) 4 and not for (la)	115
compare:	
6) 4 and eng (la)	115

Set numbers can be combined with the ''AND'' (1 and 2). Words may be combined with the ''AND'' (KIDNEY CALCULI and LITHOTRIPSY). Different steps may be taken to get the same results. Search statement 5 asks for all the articles not written in foreign languages. Search statement 6 asks for the same thing: all the articles written in English. One search (5) may be more efficient in terms of computer time.

MESH VOCABULARY

Chapter 2 covered the rules of MeSH—how indexers apply the subject headings to journal articles. As noted, the indexing for the paper index, IM, and the computer file, MEDLINE, is done simultaneously. The prospect of postcoordination is presumed by the assignment of multiple headings. Only in the computer version can the power of the postcoordination be utilized. Indexers as well as MEDLINE searchers use *Medical Subject Headings—Annotated Alphabetic List*. Figure 3.1 is a sample page from the ''M's'' that includes MYOCARDIUM. ''Annotated'' refers to the notes displayed to inform the indexer and searcher how to use the heading. Compare this to the heading shown in the Black and White MeSH in Chapter 2 (LIVER DISEASES C6.552+). There, not much more than the heading and tree number was given.

Let's look at the notes on Figure 3.1.

1. *Other Headings to Use*. A reminder about other headings that you might want to use is given first. At MYOCARDIUM, ''consider also terms at CARDIAC and HEART.'' Sometimes the abbreviation ''GEN'' for general is given. This reminds the searcher to check for the specific headings in the trees, keeping in mind the first law of indexing, namely, that articles are indexed under the most specific heading warranted by the content of the paper. MYOCARDITIS

Figure 3.1
MeSH—Annotated Alphabetical List, 1995

Myocardial Diseases
C14.280.600+

disease of myocardial tissue: differentiate from HEART DISEASES, diseases of function; for bact, parasitic & other infections of the myocardium, coord here (IM), not HEART DISEASES + infection (IM); CHAGAS CARDIOMYOPATHY is available but see note there for coords; CARDIOMYOPATHY, CONGESTIVE is also available

79; MYOCARDIAL DISEASES, PRIMARY was heading 1965–78 (Prov 1965); MYOCARDIAL DISEASES, SECONDARY was heading 1966–78

use MYOCARDIAL DISEASES to search MYOCARDIAL DISEASES, PRIMARY & MYOCARDIAL DISEASES, SECONDARY 1966–78

X Cardiomyopathies
X Myocardial Diseases, Primary
X Myocardial Diseases, Secondary
X Myocardiopathies

Myocardial Diseases, Primary see Myocardial Diseases
C14.280.600+

Myocardial Diseases, Secondary see Myocardial Diseases
C14.280.600+

Myocardial Infarction
C14.280.647.500+ C14.907.553.470.500+

do not coord with ACUTE DISEASE for "acute infarct"; DF: MYOCARDIAL INFARCT

79; was MYOCARDIAL INFARCT 1963–78

use MYOCARDIAL INFARCTION to search MYOCARDIAL INFARCT 1966–78

see related
Heart Rupture, Post-Infarction
Shoulder-Hand Syndrome
XR Infarction
XR Myocardial Ischemia

Myocardial Ischemia
C14.280.647+ C14.907.553.470+

= defic of myocard blood supply; may lead to MYOCARDIAL INFARCTION

93; HEART DISEASE, ISCHEMIC & ISCHEMIC HEART DISEASE were see CORONARY DISEASE 1969–92

use CORONARY DISEASE to search HEART DISEASE, ISCHEMIC & ISCHEMIC HEART DISEASE 1969–92

see related
Myocardial Infarction
Myocardial Reperfusion
Myocardial Revascularization
X Heart Disease, Ischemic
X Ischemia, Myocardial
X Ischemic Heart Disease

Myocardial Mitochondria see Mitochondria, Heart
A11.368.702.564.627.603 A11.904.626.627.603

Myocardial Preinfarction Syndrome see Angina, Unstable
C14.280.647.250.125.150 C14.907.553.470.250.125.150

Myocardial Reperfusion
E4.752.700.600 E5.680.730.600

note category: a technique; /adv eff permitted but consider also MYOCARDIAL REPERFUSION INJURY

89

see related
Myocardial Stunning
X Coronary Reperfusion
X Reperfusion, Myocardial
XR Myocardial Ischemia

Myocardial Reperfusion Injury
C14.280.600.615 C14.907.553.700.600
C23.814.763.530

myocardial changes after reperfusion

89

see related
Myocardial Stunning
X Reperfusion Injury, Myocardial

Myocardial Revascularization
E4.752.376.719+ E4.920.490.630+

do not use /util except by MeSH definition

73; INTERNAL MAMMARY ARTERY IMPLANTATION was heading 1975–94 (see under MYOCARDIAL REVASCULARIZATION 1975–90)

use MYOCARDIAL REVASCULARIZATION to search INTERNAL MAMMARY ARTERY IMPLANTATION 1975–94

X Internal Mammary Artery Implantation
XR Coronary Disease
XR Myocardial Ischemia

Myocardial Stimulants see Cardiotonic Agents
D18.222+

Myocardial Stunning
C14.280.647.500.375 C14.280.647.750
C14.907.553.470.500.375 C14.907.553.470.750

a type of myocardial ischemia, often caused by myocardial reperfusion

94

X Stunned Myocardium
XR Myocardial Contraction
XR Myocardial Reperfusion
XR Myocardial Reperfusion Injury

Myocardiopathies see Myocardial Diseases
C14.280.600+

Myocarditis
C14.280.600.625

inflamm of walls of heart; carditis goes here; Chagas' myocarditis = CHAGAS CARDIOMYOPATHY

Myocardium
consider also terms at CARDIAC and HEART

A2.633.580 A7.541.704
A10.690.637

the heart as tissue, differentiated from the heart as a pump (= HEART); qualif permitted: /chem /cytol /enzymol /immunol /metab /pathol /ultrastruct permitted; Manual 21.48; ischemia = MYOCARDIAL ISCHEMIA; inflammation = MYOCARDITIS; myocardial perfusion imaging, myocardial perfusion scintigraphy, myocardial imaging = HEART /radionuclide, not MYOCARDIUM /radionuclide

XR Heart

Myocardium/abnormalities see Heart Defects, Congenital
Myocardium/anatomy & histology see Heart/anatomy & histology
Myocardium/blood supply see Coronary Vessels
Myocardium/drug effects see Heart/drug effects
Myocardium/embryology see Heart/embryology
Myocardium/growth & development see Heart/growth & development
Myocardium/injuries see Heart Injuries
Myocardium/innervation see Heart/innervation
Myocardium/microbiology see Heart/microbiology
Myocardium/parasitology see Heart/parasitology
Myocardium/physiology see Heart/physiology
Myocardium/physiopathology see Heart/physiopathology
Myocardium/radiation effects see Heart/radiation effects
Myocardium/radiography see Heart/radiography
Myocardium/radionuclide imaging see Heart/radionuclide imaging
Myocardium/secretion see Heart/physiology
Myocardium/surgery see Heart Surgery
Myocardium/transplantation see Heart Transplantation
Myocardium/ultrasonography see Echocardiography

Myoclonic Epilepsy, Progressive see Epilepsy, Myoclonic
C10.228.140.490.300.280+

Myoclonic Jerking see Epilepsy, Myoclonic
C10.228.140.490.300.280+

Myoclonic Jerking, Massive see Spasms, Infantile
C10.228.140.490.300.760 F3.709.346.875

Myoclonus
C5.651.536+ C10.597.559.645
C23.888.592.574.608

a musc dis & movement disord; for "myoclonic seizure" (formerly = HYPSARRHYTHMIA) consider MYOCLONUS or EPILEPSY, MYOCLONIC or SPASMS, INFANTILE

MyoD Protein
D12.776.210.500.570.590 D12.776.260.570.590
D12.776.930.570.590

a myogenic regulatory factor controlling myogenesis

94; was MYOD FACTOR (NM) 1989–93

use MYOD PROTEIN (NM) to search MYOD FACTOR 1989–93

Myodystrophia Fetalis Deformans see Arthrogryposis
C5.550.150 C5.651.102
C5.660.77 C16.131.621.77

Myoelectric Complex, Migrating
G7.453.697.100.570 G10.261.482.570
G11.561.450.100.570

91

X Migrating Motor Complex

Myoepithelial Tumor see Myoepithelioma
C4.557.435.585

+ INDICATES THERE ARE INDENTED DESCRIPTORS IN MESH TREE STRUCTURES AT THIS NUMBER

Note: Headings appearing in bold here are capitalized in this work.

(C14.280.600.625) is a more specific heading than MYOCARDIAL DISEASES (C14.280.600+), which is more specific than HEART DISEASES (C14.280+).

2. *History Note*. Under MYOCARDIAL INFARCTION find the history notes: ''79; was MYOCARDIAL INFARCT 1963–78'' and ''use MYOCARDIAL INFARCTION to search MYOCARDIAL INFARCT 1966–78.'' This shows that MYOCARDIAL INFARCTION became the heading in 1979. Before 1979 the term in IM was MYOCARDIAL INFARCT. In this case, you may use the new term to search back to the beginning of the computerized file. The new term has been ''mapped'' back to search what the old term had covered. This is very convenient, but it is, unfortunately, not always the case. Also in this case, the change in heading is very slight. The thing to keep in mind is that the MeSH term you are looking at may not have been in use from the beginning of MEDLARS. In its various forms, MEDLINE can be searched from 1966 to the present. Earnest attempts are made to keep the MeSH searching vocabulary current with the terminology of the field, and many terms have been added, deleted, and changed over the years. Whereas in the paper index, IM, you can search only one year at a time, and the words either are or are not there on the page for that year; computer searching usually covers several years. It is necessary to know the history of a term. For example, if the term REYE'S SYNDROME became a MeSH term in 1977 and you used it to search the concept back to 1970, you may have missed a lot of information. As is often the difficulty in cases like this, the real problem is that it may not be obvious to you that you missed it. Although sometimes terms (e.g., MYOCARDIAL INFARCTION) are mapped back in time to before their introduction into the controlled vocabulary, many new terms pick up that subject only from its entry date in the system. For example, WETTING AGENTS came into the system in 1975. For 1966 to 1975, searchers need to use SURFACE-ACTIVE AGENTS. This is why the history notes are important.

3. *Precoordinated Headings and Subheadings*. Often there are directions relating to use of subheadings and precoordinated headings. The precoordinated headings take precedence over the heading-subheading combination, as we saw in Chapter 2. Therefore under MYOCARDIUM there are these directions: ''MYOCARDIUM/abnormalities see HEART DEFECTS, CONGENITAL'' and ''MYOCARDIUM/injuries see HEART INJURIES.'' The note ''qualif permitted'' lists subheadings you may use with the heading. The *Tree Number* here shows that this is from the A category, ''Anatomy.'' Overall, certain subheadings are allowed with the different categories of headings (e.g., therapies with diseases; adverse effects with chemicals). However, often a more specific direction is given at the individual heading, as seen in this case.

4. *Medical Specialties*. Reminders about medical specialty headings are helpful. CHILD PSYCHIATRY has the ''SPEC'' note: not for mental diseases (for that, use MENTAL DISORDERS). Medical specialty headings are not for the disease states. These tips are useful for paper as well as computer searching.

5. *Scope Note*. Headings sometimes have a scope note to provide direction

to meaning and usage. Under MYOCARDIUM, for example, ''the heart as tissue, differentiated from the heart as a pump (= HEART).''

6. *''See'' Refs*. The entries in smaller type direct the user to the preferred term (e.g., ''Myocardial Stimulants see Cardiotonic Agents''). In the print index, IM, the user must go to the preferred term to find the articles on that topic. On MEDLINE for the NLM system, the entry terms can be used as the search terms with the same results.

Other tools are available for the searcher. For use of MEDLINE on the NLM system, searchers need to use the *Online Services Reference Manual*. Other vendors have their own online manuals. The manual and the introductory material in the *Annotated Alphabetic List* provide important information for efficient searching. The periodicals to keep searchers updated on this system are the *NLM Technical Bulletin* and *Gratefully Yours*. Both are bimonthly NLM publications. The *NLM Technical Bulletin* includes information on changes in the MeSH vocabulary, updates on indexing practices, and news about the different NLM databases. *Gratefully Yours* was begun as a newsletter for those searching with NLM's end user software, Grateful Med; it has information for PC and Mac users of Grateful Med, testimonials on how MEDLINE searching has helped in patient care, and news of the system. One issue included, for example, the following information: ''In May, 44 percent of all journals were indexed within 30 days of receipt and 93 percent were indexed with citations available within 60 days'' (National Library of Medicine 1993a: 4). Remember that each search system has its own capabilities. PaperChase, an online vendor of MEDLINE, developed what it calls RetroMeSH. This is designed to address the problem of finding the different MeSH terms that have been used over the years to cover a concept. Where the NLM has not gone back to connect the older records to the new term, PaperChase has done so. PaperChase allows you to search with the current vocabulary and worry less about missing the older information.

SEARCHING WITH MESH ON NLM'S MEDLINE

1. *IM and NIM*. The ability to search more deeply into the topics covered by an article is available on the computer. The indexing for IM enables the searcher to find topics that are the main ideas of articles. The indexing for computer access allows retrieval also of articles that do not make it into IM under that term—NIM. The following are citation counts from MEDLINE (1991 through January 1994):

LIVER DISEASES	2710
*LIVER DISEASES	1926

There are an additional 784 articles assigned to the topic LIVER DISEASES that you will not find in IM. Remember, an article may have ten to fifteen MeSH headings, but perhaps two to five will be designated IM. In the NLM system, use an asterisk to limit yourself to those articles with the main ideas.

2. *Explosions.* Along with the Boolean "AND," the Explosion (EXP) facility effectively utilizes the great power of the computer. Indexing specificity has been looked at several times. As searchers, however, we often want to retrieve both the general and the specifics for a parameter of a search. An Explosion is a grand "ORing" device. Let's say we want to find articles on liver diseases. We look up the term in the *Annotated Alphabetic*. The term is there with its *Tree Number*, C6.552+. The *Tree Structure* is checked at C6.552 and more specific entries are found. (See Chapter 2 for part of that Tree.) What to do? We can "OR" all the terms together:

LIVER DISEASES or ACUTE YELLOW ATROPHY or CHOLESTASIS INTRAHEPATIC or ALAGILLE SYNDROME or LIVER CIRRHOSIS, BILIARY or FATTY LIVER or FATTY LIVER, ALCOHOLIC or etc.

This is time consuming and burdensome, not to mention that people will make mistakes in typing. This is where the Explode (EXP) command is so handy.

LIVER DISEASES	2710
but - exp LIVER DISEASES	19,484

All the terms indented under LIVER DISEASES were "ORed" with LIVER DISEASES to get the total of 19,484. You may combine the capability of main ideas and Explosions.

exp*LIVER DISEASES 15,590

For very large categories that would be exploded often, the system offers Pre-explosions (PX). The system gathers the posting together for you ahead of time.

DIGESTIVE SYSTEM DISEASES (px) 66,213

3. *Trees.* There is a convenient command here that lets you see the *Tree Structures* online. "Tree HEPATITIS" gives the following display.

LIVER DISEASES	C6.552
HEPATITIS	C6.552.380
HEPATITIS, ALCOHOLIC	C6.552.380.290
HEPATITIS, ANIMAL	C6.552.380.315 (+)
HEPATITIS, TOXIC	C6.552.380.615
HEPATITIS, VIRAL, HUMAN	C6.552.380.705 (+)

The "+," as usual, signals more narrower terms. If you do a "Tree" command with "HEPATITIS, VIRAL, HUMAN," the HEPATITIS A, HEPATITIS B, and more terms are displayed.

4. *Free Text Searching*. In Chapter 2, a controlled vocabulary thesaurus–based index (IM) was compared with a natural language index (BA). The computer searching lets you use both the controlled vocabulary of IM and the free text of BA. MEDLINE retains its controlled vocabulary, MeSH, on the computer and offers searching on the words in the title and abstract (TW). The consistency of a controlled vocabulary and the flexibility of free text is there to be utilized.

HEPATITIS (MH)	511
hepatitis (TW)	9554

In this case, many more citations have "hepatitis" in the title or abstract than have HEPATITIS as the assigned MeSH heading. We may presume that in some of these articles hepatitis is mentioned only peripherally and does not warrant inclusion as an NIM term. In many other cases, the article may have been indexed under a more specific term (e.g., HEPATITIS A). We would therefore not have picked it up in the 511 articles. Remember, the broad and the narrow apply here, too.

HEPATITIS	511
exp HEPATITIS	7069

5. *Subheadings*. Topical subheadings are often assigned with the MeSH headings. Effective searching with subheadings takes some skill and understanding. It is also good to remember the warning from Funk and Reid (1983), cited in Chapter 2: Subheadings are susceptible more than other parts of MeSH to varying judgments by the indexers. Also, just as the MeSH headings are arranged hierarchically in the trees and are assigned by relevant specificity, subheadings are hierarchical, too. "Therapy" is assigned as a subheading to a disease if the treatment is not covered by one of the more specific "therapy" subheadings. Specific subheadings under "therapy" include

—diet therapy

—drug therapy

—nursing

—prevention & control

—radiotherapy

—surgery

  transplantation [as a narrower term under "surgery"]

For example, if the article is about drug therapy of hepatitis, you find the article under HEPATITIS/dt, not under HEPATITIS/th. The slash followed by a two-letter abbreviation is a way to enter a subheading. The heading with subheading combination may also be entered as a main idea (IM). The article needs to appear under the subheading ''drug therapy'' under the MeSH heading HEPATITIS in *Index Medicus* when you enter it this way:

*HEPATITIS/dt	10

The subheading may also be included in an Explosion.

exp* HEPATITIS/dt	345
exp*HEPATITIS/dt	213

If you wish to retrieve that MeSH heading with more than one subheading, another command can be used. The following picks up HEPATITIS/dt or HEPATITIS/dh or HEPATITIS/su:

Subheadings apply dt,dh,su	
HEPATITIS	46
Subheadings cancel	

Another way to search for subheadings is possible. Wanting to make your search a little broader and unsure about the application of subheadings, you may choose to search in a free-floating mode. Search with the Boolean ''AND'' just as if the subheadings were MeSH headings. Doing this does not link the subheading with one MeSH heading, so the procedure is not as precise. But it will pick up an article if one of the assigned MeSH headings has that subheading attached to it.

HEPATITIS and dt (sh)	57
*HEPATITIS and dt (sh)	44
exp HEPATITIS and dt (sh)	588
exp*HEPATITIS and dt (sh)	484

The capability of Exploding the subheadings became available to searchers in 1991. This capability is used with the free-floating method of searching subheadings.

HEPATITIS and th& (px)	142
exp HEPATITIS and th& (px)	2640

Using the free-floating technique picks up those specific subheadings under ''therapy'' noted above: diet therapy, drug therapy, nursing, prevention & control, radiotherapy, surgery, and transplantation.

FILE MESH

The NLM system contains several other databases in addition to MEDLINE. One database is the computer counterpart to MeSH. To move to that database, type in ''File MeSH.'' The searcher can consult this instead of the printed volumes for information on allowable subheadings with the heading, scope note, references to related descriptors, Tree Numbers, history, and so on. Also available is information about the number of citations with that term made over the years. The bibliographic database of MEDLINE is available to 1966, but NLM searching is done in segments of years. Therefore, in the MeSH file you can see the number of postings for the term in each segment. Consider for example, the display for HEPATITIS (covering 1966 through January 1994):

MED—511	MED is 1991–January 1994
MED—*300	
M89—394	M89 is 1989–1990
M89—*277	
M85—813	M85 is 1985–1988
M85—*451	
M80—1670	M80 is 1980–1984
M80—*932	
M75—2350	M75 is 1975–1979
M75—*1264	
M66—4572	M66 is 1966–1974
M66—*2331	

There are two entries for each segment. These represent the total number of citations and the part of that number that is IM (main idea of an article). Also, note that there are larger groups of years earlier on (M66 covers 1966–1974). Not until the mid-1970s did abstracts start to be included. Once they were, the individual records took up more storage space. Thus post-1974 groupings contain fewer years.

SUBJECTS AND THE SEARCHER'S STRATEGY

''Searching With MeSH on NLM's MEDLINE'' showed us that there are many variations to choose from when searching for information on a topic. Subject searching involves a good bit of discretion on the part of the searcher, who must continuously make choices. Although there are many rules to understand, good searchers often retrieve different results from the same search request. It might be admitted that searching is more of an art than a science. We do know, however, that many users of the system either are oblivious to MeSH or simply do not bother to use the database. They stick with the free text searching, typing whatever words they associate with the concept. In fact, many databases do not have controlled vocabularies, and the only way to search them is to use free text. This should be kept in mind when we evaluate or use the systems. Take, for example, the UnCover database that is the table of contents of thousands of journal articles covering the spectrum of topics in a library. Let's say that the searcher is using it to look for information on mental disorders of professional athletes. We may search for ''mental disorders'' and ''professional athletes.'' However, what happens if the article is about ''baseball players'' and ''schizophrenia''? Vocabulary control is not a trivial issue.

UNIT RECORD: SEARCHABLE FIELDS

So far we have looked at subject searching with the use of MeSH, and in the NLM system that is the default field. No category qualification is needed with entering a MeSH term. However, there are other ways to search the system. If a word that is not a MeSH term is entered without a category qualifier, the system checks the MeSH file and comes back with a No Postings report. This is unlike the searching of MEDLINE on other systems. On Ovid Technologies, for example, an unqualified word is automatically searched in the MeSH field, the title word field, and the abstract word field. To search for a word from the title or abstract on NLM, the category qualifier for text word (TW) is needed (as we saw with ''hepatitis'' earlier). The text word search covers the words in the title and abstract. The (TF) is the qualifier for searching for title words only. This acts as a great supplement for subject searches. There are a lot of MeSH terms—over 17,000—but they cannot be as specific or up to date as an author's terminology. Going from print to computer not only adds the great power of Boolean searching and Explosions but also increases the searchable database. Consult NLM's *Online Services Reference Manual* for more information on searching MEDLINE and the other databases. Each database has a unit record, which displays the searchable fields. To search for an author, for example, use (AU). Let's say that you are looking for an author whose last name is Rice and first initial is *S*, but you do not know the middle initial.

rice s (au)	3
rice s: (au)	14

The colon (:) is the truncation symbol in the NLM system. It can take the place of one or zero or many characters. The symbol for one wildcard character is the number sign (#). It is convenient for retrieving both the singular and the plural (e.g., eye#). To see an alphabetical display and postings statements, use the neighbor (NBR) command. This lists the entries in alphabetical order. You can then select (sel) from the choices shown:

NBR rice s (au)	
1) RICE RR JR	3
2) RICE RT	4
3) RICE S	3
4) RICE SA	7
5) RICE SJ	2
6) RICE SM	1
7) RICE SQ	1
8) RICE T	29
sel 3–7	14

We have already discussed a few of the commands of the system: tree, file, subheadings, and neighbor. The print command is probably the most used. The prompt for user interaction is ss#/c?. The ''ss#'' is for search statement number and ''c'' is for command. The print command is used to display the citations and parts of the unit record that have been retrieved. (The unit record, recall, lists the fields in that database.) Type in ''prt'' and the most recently added citations will be displayed with the author, title, and source fields along with the unique identifying number for that citation. Tailored prt commands can also be given for the fields in the unit record. For example, ''prt ti, ab, la, mh'' will yield the title, abstract, language, and medical subject headings. To find more information about the print command (as well as to request other help) use the command ''Explain.'' ''Explain Print'' gives information on how to display the different fields and records in a set.

COMPUTER MANIPULATION OF BIBLIOGRAPHIC DATA

Behind the scenes, combinations of parameters for thousands of journal article citations and abstracts are manipulated by the computer system. How does the system handle such a large database so quickly? The database is constructed from three files (see Figure 3.2, which comes from the *Online Services Reference Manual*). The Index File alphabetically arranges all the terms in the database: subject headings, authors, title words, and so on. Each index entry in the Index File has a record of the number of citations containing it in the database as well as the classification of its field type (e.g., author). It also has a number that links it to the Postings File. The Postings File for that entry has a record of the citation

Figure 3.2
Internal Computer Files

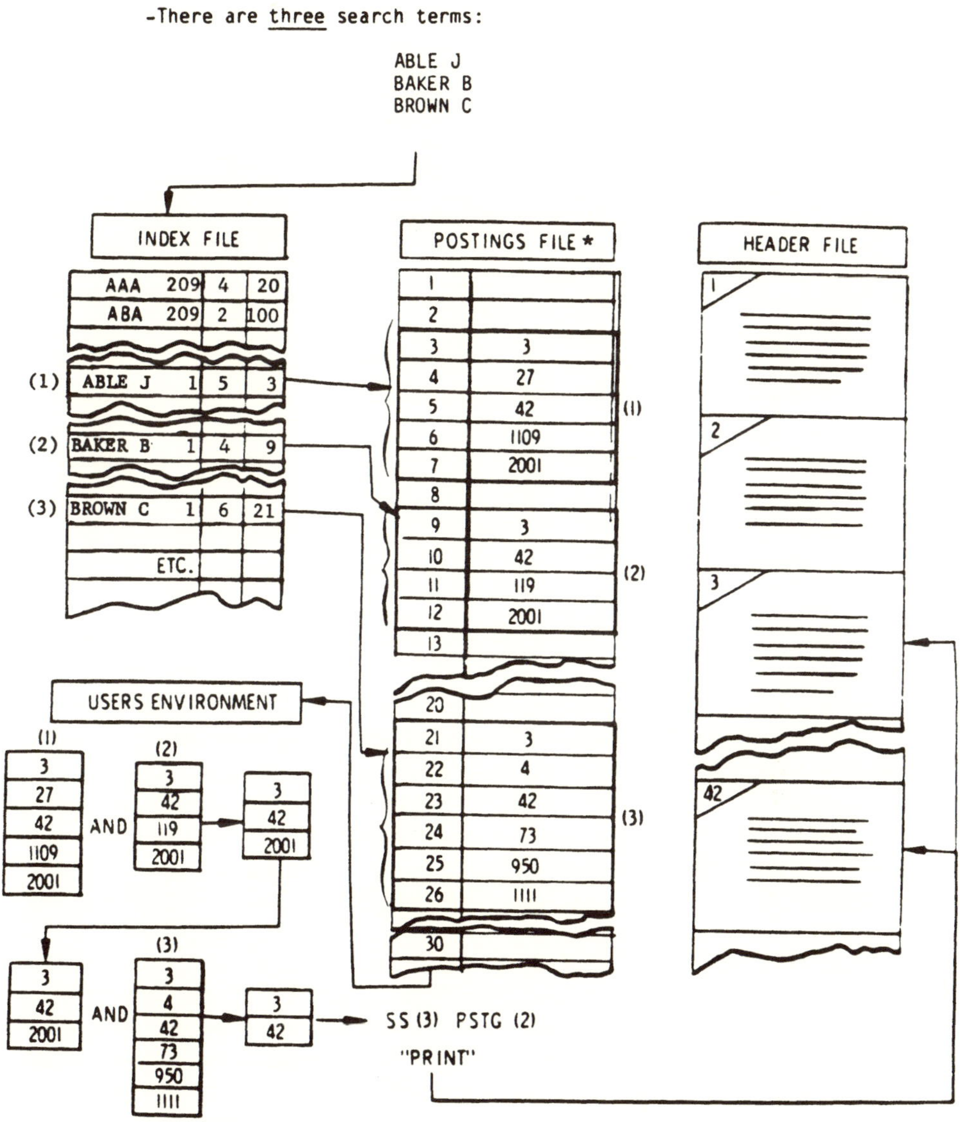

*The CAN Numbers are really very long, two-part numbers, for example, 7003394 (109428/2). The short, simplified numbers used here are for purposes of illustration.

Source: Online Services Reference Manual, 1988.

numbers. Those citation numbers take you to the Header File, which contains the full record for each citation. Searching records (i.e., citations) directly in the Header File would be like some word processing searches: You would be matching character strings sequentially through the full text. Doing this would take a great deal of time in a very big file like MEDLINE. Searching efficiency in these bibliographic databases is not based on the string of characters you are searching but on the index file. Another name for the index file is the inverted file.

BEYOND NLM: SEARCHING MEDLINE ON DIFFERENT SYSTEMS

To reiterate, the different online as well as CD-ROM vendors of MEDLINE all get the database from the same source—NLM. They all lease the same database. Given the same years, the MEDLINE database on each of these systems is identical. If, however, you key in the same words on different vendors, your results will usually not be the same. Why is that? Here is a search limited to one year, 1992, on three versions of MEDLINE: NLM, CDP Online (Ovid Technologies), and SilverPlatter CD-ROM.

HEPATITIS (NLM)	224
HEPATITIS (CDP)	3697
HEPATITIS (SilverPlatter)	2385

When words are entered into NLM's MEDLINE, they are checked against the MeSH vocabulary. Unless the user qualifies the input to another field, the default field is MeSH. The user can stipulate that he or she is directing the search to the title and abstract words or direct it to any other searchable part of the unit record. For instance, he or she can type in ''hepatitis (au)'' or ''hepatitis (tw).'' When a word is typed into other versions of searching software (Ovid and SilverPlatter in these examples), that word is automatically checked in the MeSH vocabulary plus other fields. For those systems, the searching of the MeSH fields will find a match if it is the exact descriptor (e.g., HEPATITIS) or also part of the descriptor (e.g., HEPATITIS A). (In 1991, NLM introduced a way to search a word within a descriptor—MeSH Heading Fragment, or MHF.) The most obvious other fields are title and abstract. The searcher may also designate in the different systems which field he or she does or does not want to search. The point is that because the searching software varies for the different systems, the unwary searcher will get different results with each system. You need to know the database and its structure. Also, you need to understand the particulars of the system you are using. There are real differences and advantages for the various systems (Hunter 1991). These aspects of the systems are going to change. For several years the NLM version of MEDLINE offered the three basic Boolean operators: "AND," "OR," and "AND NOT." There was no provision for a full database search of adjacent terms in a title or abstract. NLM did offer a string search capability, but that was practical only for a selected set of a few hundred citations. Your search would have to have gotten you to that point first before an adjacency could be used. Meanwhile services like BRS (CDP, Ovid) and DIALOG have offered that searching technique for quite a while. Here is an example. You want to find articles using HL-60 cells in the experiment. It is not a MeSH term and there is no MeSH term specific enough. You would like to search HL60, HL-60, plus HL adj 60. On OVID, doing this is no problem. On NLM, it has been not as simple to do. Not until 1995 was a full adjacency feature added to the NLM system (National Library of Medicine 1995b).

SEARCH STRATEGY AND TIPS FOR GOOD SEARCHING

Three requirements for a successful search include knowing the vocabulary, knowing the capabilities of the search system and database, and obtaining an understanding of the request to fit it into a Boolean search. A fourth requirement can be added: Know your requestor. This will help you a great deal with requirement three. Much has been written about the characteristics that make people good or not so good searchers. Personal qualities like intelligence and perseverance are mentioned. Experience is also often noted. Nothing is going to be added here along that line. One variable that usually makes a big impact on the success of the search is simply the topic of the search. Many subjects fit easily into the artificial mechanics of Boolean searches. Many others do not. Some topics can be described in concrete terms that match the vocabulary with little chance for multiple meanings. Other topics seem more vague. You might say this, that your job as a reference librarian is to ask those questions, clarify the request, and pin down the patron to specify exactly what he or she wants. Some topics, however, remain difficult to squeeze into the vocabulary and the Boolean search.

During instruction in online searching, there has often been great emphasis placed on doing detailed planning before going online. Often, online time is a major cost factor for database use. The relatively low cost of MEDLINE has made this argument less compelling. The searcher has logged on, quickly entered the terms, printed a few citations online or offline, and logged off. The batch searches of NLM in the 1960s have been relived hundreds of thousands of times throughout the years across the country. In the constant effort to defeat that ticking clock and the accumulating cost, the searchers have abandoned one of the greatest strengths of computer searching—interaction. The feedback that you get online from the initial results is a valuable guide. If the requestor can be there during the session, so much the better. The search will take longer, especially if the requestor is there making comments and suggestions, but the outcome will usually be more satisfactory to all parties.

PRECISION AND RECALL

At times you are satisfied retrieving a few relevant citations and not concerned about other useful articles that are missed. This brings up the topics of precision and recall. In the early 1960s, large-scale experiments were conducted on information storage and retrieval in Cranfield, England. The projects were intended to characterize the efficiency of the use of natural language versus controlled vocabularies in retrieving information. The head of these projects was C. W. Cleverdon. To calculate outcomes and make comparisons, Cleverdon and his colleagues devised two measures: precision and recall. In library science, few things can be meaningfully quantified. For recall and precision, at least, numbers can be determined. Let's say you are looking for articles on aspects of hepatitis. You enter your search and get 100 citations. After examining the 100 citations, 30 are determined to be relevant. Because 30 out of 100 were on target, precision for the search is 30%. In some way a count has been done of the whole database. This would not be easy in a large database. In fact, it is impossible. Out of the database that may contain tens of thousands or hundreds of thousands of citations, for example, it is determined somehow that 300 articles talk about your aspect of hepatitis. You retrieved 30. Because 30 out of 300 is 10%, your recall is 10%. To enlarge your recall and retrieve more of the rest of the 270 articles you missed, you will decrease the precision from 30%. Raising the 30% precision probably would yield a smaller than 10% recall. An inverse relationship is typically found. There is a way to cut down on false drops, but the price is lower recall. Ways to lower the number of false drops and increase precision include limiting the search to main ideas (IM) and to ideas stated in the title. Enlarging recall can be achieved by doing the reverse. Use NIM, pick up terms from the abstract or even from full-text databases, enter "OR" to find more terms, and do more Explosions. You will decide in which direction to take the search on the basis of the needs of the requestor.

HOW TO FIND THE GOOD ARTICLES

There are many techniques to try in searching the literature for the subjects that you are interested in. The idea of the quality of the literature search has been bound up with the capacity to get information on the topic and, perhaps, to avoid getting information that is not meaningful for the question at hand. Let us say that that part has been successful. We have gotten a substantial number of articles that address our topic. Is there a technique for us to pull the "good" articles out of these? Chapter 1 included information that shows that not all biomedical journals are equal and not all journal articles are the same quality. One piece of evidence we saw used the citation history of a publication. This might be one way of approaching a quality judgment. However, we are often searching the most recent literature, and the citation history results are not in.

One device that may be used in MEDLINE for this purpose is the review article. The primary journal literature has the purpose of reporting new findings from biomedical research. Review articles are written by scientists in the field for the purpose of bringing together the findings of those primary journal articles. A review article may evaluate just a handful of articles but often includes dozens or even hundreds. On MEDLINE, the searcher may limit the results by requesting only review articles on that topic. In 1988 NLM enlarged its categories of review articles. Before that, the designation REVIEW was for a review of the current literature. Then, REVIEW, ACADEMIC; REVIEW LITERATURE; REVIEW, MULTICASE; REVIEW OF REPORTED CASES; and REVIEW, TUTORIAL became terms (Snow 1989). To retrieve any type of review, use REVIEW. However, if you are not a specialist in the subject in question and would like an introduction to it and its recent literature, use REVIEW, TUTORIAL. The thorough and critical reviews of the current literature can be found with REVIEW, ACADEMIC.

The review article may be useful, but other techniques are needed. R. Brian Haynes and his colleagues at McMaster University have investigated and written about the process of finding the ''good'' clinical articles. In particular, there was a series of their articles in the *Annals of Internal Medicine* (Haynes et al. 1986), ''How to Keep up with the Medical Literature,'' and a more recent series (Oxman, Sackett, and Guyatt 1993) in *JAMA*, ''Users' Guide to the Medical Literature.'' In 1991 the indexers at MEDLARS initiated a major change in the use of publication types for journal articles. Each edition of the *Annotated Alphabetic List* since then has a section on publication types. This new classification opened up another way to find ''good'' articles.

Because the main purpose of this whole endeavor is to get new, useful information into the hands of primary care health professionals when they are treating their patients, often the need is for ''good'' clinical articles. That is, the health care providers need information not on studies with rats or just test tube results (Haynes 1990; Lindberg et al. 1993). They need information that can be used with their patients now. Many articles retrieved from a typical MEDLINE search do not present information ready for clinical care. It has always been difficult in the past to request articles on a topic that were just ''clinical.'' Here is where the section on publication types can be used to limit the search, to find the clinical articles. One publication type is CLINICAL TRIAL, ''Pre-planned, usually controlled, clinical study of the safety, efficacy, or optimum dosage schedule of one or more diagnostic, therapeutic, or prophylactic drugs, devices, or techniques in humans selected according to predetermined criteria of eligibility and observed for predefined evidence of favorable and unfavorable effects'' (National Library of Medicine1994b, I-18). In addition, an indication of the type of methodology and population treated would also be helpful. In Chapter 1, in Dr. Wolff's experiment with his patients the term ''double blind'' was used. Dr. Wolff did not know which patients were getting the drug in question and neither did the patients. To locate this study, the searcher can use the MeSH heading DOUBLE-BLIND METHOD. Consider also the publication type RANDOMIZED CONTROLLED TRIAL. Other publication types of interest here are META-ANALYSIS, MULTICENTER STUDY, CONSENSUS DEVELOPMENT CONFERENCE, CONTROLLED CLINICAL TRIAL, and PRACTICE GUIDELINE, as well as the various phases of the clinical trial (e.g., CLINICAL TRIAL, PHASE III). There are actually two reasons for these publication types. They should help clinicians identify useful information. Also, publication types can be utilized in searching for issues of cost, quality, and management of care. Is there literature on how the physician should be treating the patient for the ailment in question? This involves the cost of care as well as the quality of care. This issue will come up again in Chapter 7. Here is the description of PRACTICE GUIDELINE: "A set of directions or principles to assist the health care practitioner with patient care decisions about appropriate diagnostic, therapeutic, or other clinical procedures for specific clinical circumstances" (National Library of Medicine 1994b, I-24).

One distinction needs to be noted here. There may exist a MeSH heading that is close to the publication type (e.g., RANDOMIZED CONTROLLED TRIALS). The MeSH heading is used for articles that discuss that idea (e.g., a discussion about the use or dependability of randomized controlled trials). The publication type RANDOMIZED CONTROLLED TRIAL is a description of the methodology of the article in hand. An attempt to help physicians and other health care providers get at the articles that they can use, these devices represent an important tool for them to use in handling the literature.

A pair of other publication types are designed to warn MEDLINE searchers about articles. This is something uniquely suited to the computer. There are occasions when the publisher or the authors of a study find that some work that they have done contains an error that may render the findings invalid. Publishers sometimes send out errata to subscribers, and libraries may put those errata in with the original article. When you look in your copies of IM, however, you will not find notes at those citations warning you about the entry. NLM does not recall the volumes to "repair" them. However, on the computer, there is something that can be done. The article that announces the retraction is indexed for MEDLINE with the publication type RETRACTION OF PUBLICATION. In addition, the original citation pulled up in a search has a note in the title indicating that it has been retracted by the later journal citation and has been assigned the publication type RETRACTED PUBLICATION. The searcher could come across the retraction either at the retracting article or at the original (retracted) article.

IS MEDLINE THE BEST OF ALL WORLDS?

Medical libraries have had a good deal with MEDLINE. It is a large and well-constructed database. The MeSH vocabulary may be the best searching vocabulary around. The indexers are well trained. The capability to get the specific or the general or both with the Explode command gives us flexibility and power. The topics requested are generally fairly concrete in the biomedical field. This is not to say that everybody uses the same words to refer to the same thing, but it seems to be a better situation than with the social sciences or humanities. MEDLINE has always been cheap. Fifteen to thirty dollars per hour compares very favorably to the dollar-a-minute physical sciences databases and the two-dollars-per-minute business databases and the three-dollars-or-more-per-minute legal databases. In addition, our users often have grants and contracts to charge their searches to. Compare that to the old charge of $70 per hour for Philosopher's Index. Searchers of medical databases had a big advantage in the 1970s and 1980s.

CD-ROM: DEATH OF THE CLOCK

We have not left the online era. However, alternatives to access have appeared that let us approach searching in a different way. Organizations can lease tapes from database producers and mount them on their own local computer. The cost is not usually trivial, but the mentality of using the sources goes back to the unhurried days before we were charged by the time being used. A subscription to CA might cost $16,000 per year in print, but it was available for however much use hundreds of patrons might make of it. Locally mounted databases and CD-ROMs give us back our old comfortable ways. Linger and browse. Experiment. Drift through the citations as you might wander through the stacks. Again, the cost of the CD-ROMs is now not insignificant. However, the charge cannot be measured just in searching style. Making the indexes convenient and easy opens them up to much larger audiences. Online was intimidating for many years. You not only had to pay for it but also had no assurance that you would be happy with what you purchased. You also often had to deal with a librarian. Even if you liked librarians, it was still not that convenient to do the search only when you could arrange it with the librarian.

Local access has meant that the service is now much more widely used. Online searching had a tremendous impact on interlibrary loan. Local access does also. And this local access means as well that the literature in general is being used much more than it was. Your collection is being used more. If our reason for having a library and being librarians is to facilitate the use of information, the CD-ROM and its cousins have been a great help in fulfilling our mission.

END USER SEARCHING, GRATEFUL MED, AND UMLS

The topic of end user searching has been around for a while. Individuals have had the opportunity to get passwords and documentation from vendors for many years. There have even been menu-driven searching for quite some time. Now, however, it is easier. Software is available to log on, upload a search, download a search, and place the citations in a file in a database of your own in your computer or on your disk. And, of course, CD-ROMs can do away with the complication of arranging for your own equipment if you would like to use the library's workstation or network. A question you may have is this: If searching has become this easy, why do I, the librarian, need to be concerned with arcane notions of fields and vocabulary control? Two reasons. You will still be called upon to perform effective searches. Second, you can help the end users perform better searches. When CD-ROMs and Online Public Access Catalogs (OPACs) are introduced into the library, the patrons find them terrific and take to them right away. Just because a CD-ROM is easy to use, however, does not mean that patrons are getting what they could or what they need. Your help is needed in instruction. Remember the debate in libraries or library schools: Do I give them the information or do I show them how to get the information so they can do it themselves? However you might think of that philosophically, you can provide a great service in end user searching by providing the latter. This goes right to the heart of the message to physicians and others to master the means of being lifelong learners.

Much of the software available today was developed with the end user in mind. Grateful Med is the software available from NLM designed to take the physician-searcher through the whole searching process with a menu interface. It is inexpensive, and improved editions have come out annually. Note that there are many software packages from private companies around as well. Other NLM innovations address the problems of subject searching in their databases. The UMLS (Unified Medical Language System) was mentioned in Chapter 2. This project has attempted to understand various terminologies used in medicine and then to form links among the terms. Its goal has been to construct from these links a device to aid the health care professional as searcher. First NLM researchers gathered up all the words in medicine that they could find from the various vocabularies: *Medical Subject Headings* (NLM), *Library of Congress Subject Headings* (LC), *Current Procedural Terminology* (AMA), *International Classification of Diseases* (World Health Organization), *Systemized Nomenclature of Medicine* (College of American Pathologists), and *Diagnostic and Statistical Manual* (American Psychiatric Association). This developed into what was named a *Metathesaurus.* Another step was to determine the relationships among the terms; so NLM researchers devised the ''Semantic Network.'' The purpose of doing this was to enable the searchers to enter any word they associate with that subject and have the program automatically translate it into what the system uses for that subject. The computer program that has been in the testing phase is ''Coach'' (Kingsland et al. 1993). The plan for the coming Internet application of Grateful Med includes this type of searching program.

NATURAL LANGUAGE SEARCHING

We would really like to enable the searcher to enter a search request in natural language. Sometimes the phrase ''natural language,'' is used synonymously with ''free text,'' discussed earlier. This type of searching, you will recall, does not use ''controlled vocabulary.'' Here, ''natural language searching'' refers to something different—the use of plain, English sentences (e.g., ''Is marijuana helpful in alleviating some side effects of cancer treatment?''). Actually, some systems are starting to use natural language. Ovid and Aries Systems do offer the option to enter your search in that form. This type of searching may be even more attractive for use with a full-text database. Westlaw, a vendor of databases covering the law, has implemented this with Westlaw Is Natural (WIN) (Pritchard-Schoh 1993). This system takes the input of sentences or phrases, removes the trivial words such as ''the,'' performs a truncation on the remaining words to pull up plurals and variants, and compares those words to the words in the database. That comparison looks at the frequency of those words in the document and in the database. That analysis is then used to rank the documents in the database for their relevancy to the question. This type of research with frequency analysis and weighting has been going on in library and information science for many years. Now there are products that have left the test stage and are used by our patrons and us. On the Internet, too, these devices are available (e.g., WAIS, or Wide Area Information Servers). Web search engines with increasing power are being developed so quickly that singling them out here is of little value.

These two systems, WIN and WAIS, use a very different type of searching mechanism than our traditional Boolean. Search terms are ''ORed'' in these systems. In the parenthetical example above, documents would be found with the most occurrences of ''marijuana,'' ''cancer,'' ''alleviating,'' ''side,'' and the like. The publications found are ranked by relevance, and the highest-ranked publications are displayed to the searcher first. This is really very different from what we have been doing. Let us see what happens with the Boolean search and with the relevancy weighting search. We will use four parameters:

cancer
marijuana
therapy
side effects

The Boolean search is like this:

cancer and marijuana and therapy and side effects

Any citation that you retrieve has to have all four parameters in it. Citations with just ''cancer'' are not retrieved. Citations with just ''cancer'' and ''marijuana'' are not retrieved. Citations with just ''cancer'' and ''marijuana'' and ''therapy'' are not retrieved. You never see any of these whether they have zero or one or two or three of the parameters.

What happens with relevancy searching: cancer or marijuana or therapy or side effects? The retrieved articles do not have to have all four parameters. The search is based upon ''OR,'' not ''AND.'' This does not, intuitively, make sense. However, the retrieval is based on weighting. If a record (i.e., citation of an article or full text of the article) has eight occurrences of ''cancer'' and fifteen occurrences of ''marijuana,'' it will be ranked higher than an article with three occurrences of ''cancer'' and four occurrences of ''marijuana.'' This is a simplification of what happens. The key thing searchers must remember is that the retrieved citations do not have to include all the parameters. Some applications enable searchers to ''force'' the system to include parameters (e.g., an article has to have ''marijuana'' in it to be retrieved).

This ''smart'' searching system enables the searcher to work with a text that has not been previously analyzed, cataloged, or indexed. A traditional thesaurus may be utilized in the program to bring together the ''cancer'' terms and the ''neoplasm'' terms. However, the processing is done on the searching end. This is similar to searching the free text databases such as BIOSIS but has a much more potent search engine. Why is this type of natural language searching in demand? As we look to all the databases becoming available via the Internet, can we really provide the type of indexing that has been done on those abstracting and indexing services? It seems impossible. Therefore instead of indexing, we are utilizing these ''smart'' searching programs. Do we lose precision when we rely on the natural language search engines? ''So far, almost everyone who has compared Boolean searching with the new non-Boolean searching finds that each retrieves relevant documents. Searchers hoping for comprehensive results should use both'' (Tenopir 1994, 36). Pritchard-Schoh (1993) found the same thing. Both types of searches retrieve relevant items, but often the two sets contain different relevant items. This gives us, as searchers, pause. If we examine citation searching, we will see that it often retrieves relevant items different than those retrieved by subject word searching. In a way, this new relevancy searching and the citation searching have something in common. They are tools that end users will use. Boolean searching with its ''AND,'' ''OR,'' ''NOT,'' ''ADJ,'' and so on, may not be intuitive to people, and end users have generally not been interested in learning it.

It would likewise be convenient if the full text of databases across many disciplines could be searched with the same software in one place. Such standardization describes LEXIS-NEXIS. The full text of many newspapers, magazines, laws, regulations, and abstracting and indexing services, including MEDLINE, are in it. This question must be asked, then: If there are these sophisticated programs to utilize to search the literature, do we really need to know the details that go on behind the scenes as suggested in this chapter? Perhaps we don't need to find and use the most primitive version of a system and only rely on it; but for now, at least, we do need to understand the workings of the system in order to understand what we have and have not gotten—and what we have yet to get.

POSTSCRIPT ON POSTCOORDINATION

The precoordinated subject headings often used in the *Library of Congress Subject Headings* serve a useful purpose (e.g., Medicine and the Humanities; Nurses in Television; Imaging Systems in Biology). They represent guesses by librarians as to what combinations of ideas people will find usefully grouped together. However, precoordinated headings offer a limited view of the world. A vocabulary of subject headings can include only a relatively small number of these combinations. Putting the power of "AND" in the user's hand makes possible a seemingly infinite number of combinations. The widespread use of computers has brought the power of Boolean searching to many. Another aspect was stated this way: "Pre-coordinate terms in a print index express the indexer's certainty; post-coordinate terms in an electronic index express the index user's hopes" (Preschel 1989: 55). Precoordinated terms are assigned with the publication in hand. This not only guarantees that the ideas will appear together but also often prescribes the relationship among the words (e.g., "Nutritionally Induced Diseases"). In postcoordination, there is the possibility that the words will appear together but not as assumed. "Neck" and "Pain" may find information about discomfort in the neck. They may also find the idiom "pain in the neck." "Cancer" and "Marijuana" may yield articles exactly on target about the use of marijuana to alleviate the pain of cancer therapy. Postcoordination may also enable the searcher to retrieve citations about patients with cancer who also happen to be smoking marijuana or individuals who have taken up smoking marijuana as a reaction to a family member's diagnosis of cancer. Postcoordination may result in false drops. The only given is that the two or more terms are present in the record of the document. Proximity operators help here. The user can require that the two words be physically next to each other in a particular order. This helps. You can distinguish between "Library School" and the "School Library," for example. The devices for weighting terms and displaying records in the order of proposed relevance are more attempts to get beyond the limitations of the regular "AND." We will hope for advances in the research from linguistics, automatic indexing, artificial intelligence, neural networks, expert systems, and the like.

While we utilize what is available to us as well as wait for more advanced techniques, here is a word in support of the Boolean "AND." The use of "AND" brings with it the capability of bringing ideas together that no one else may have thought of before. Don Swanson (1986) has written on this. One case he brought up talked about the literature on Raynaud's disease and the literature on dietary fish oils. The Raynaud's literature mentioned elevated blood viscosity. The literature on dietary fish oils gave information on their effect of reducing blood viscosity. Swanson found it instructive that the two literatures were separate. They did not appear in the same journals, they did not cite each other, nor did they cite any other articles in common. Clearly, searching the literature can be a research endeavor itself, making connections that have not been thought of before. In fact, a few years after Swanson proposed this connection, it was field tested, and dietary fish oils were found to be useful in treating Raynaud's disease.

BEYOND MEDLINE: OTHER BIOMEDICAL DATABASES

At the beginning of this chapter, it was stated that you will become an expert in MEDLINE and that you need to be aware of other resources (Brandsma et al. 1990; Tilley 1990). The list that follows indicates some of those other resources, mostly in the bibliographic realm. Here are included: (1) other databases available on the National Library of Medicine system and (2) databases on two traditional library vendors (a listing from Ovid and DIALOG). Some brief notes are attached. More nonbibliographic databases on the Internet will be looked at in Chapters 5 and 6.

1. *National Library of Medicine*:

AIDSDRUGS (drugs being tested in AIDS clinical trials)

AIDSLINE (bibliographic citations on AIDS from many publication types)

AIDSTRIALS (descriptions of individual clinical trials on AIDS)

AVLINE (citations to audiovisuals and computer software)

BIOETHICSLINE (citations from many types of publications on ethical and legal issues in biomedicine)

BIOTECHSEEK (journal biotechnology citations not in MEDLINE)

CANCERLIT (citations on cancer from many publication types; this topic, more comprehensive than MEDLINE)

CATLINE (cataloging records, primarily for books)

CHEMLINE (chemical names)

DENTALPROJ (descriptions of ongoing research projects in dentistry)

DIRLINE (directory of organizations providing information services)

HEALTH (Health Planning and Administration database noted in Chapter 2)

HISTLINE (publications starting in 1964 on the history of medicine)

HSTAR (health services research to be covered in Chapters 4 and 7)

PDQ—Physician Data Query (cancer protocols and directory of physicians)

POPLINE (citations from many publication types on family planning and demographics)

SERLINE (information on serial titles in the NLM collection)

SPACELINE (bibliographic citations to many types of publications on space life sciences research)

TOXLINE (citations from many publication types on toxicology)

Along with ELHILL, NLM also has another computer system, TOXNET (Toxicology Data Network), which includes the following databases on toxic and hazardous substances:

Chemical Carcinogenesis Research Information System (CCRIS)

Developmental and Reproductive Toxicology (DART)

Environmental Mutagen Information Center (EMIC)

Environmental Teratology Information Center Backfile (ETICBACK)

Gene-Tox (for genetic toxicology)

Hazardous Substances Data Bank (HSDB)

Integrated Risk Information System (IRIS)

Registry of Toxic Effects of Chemical Substances (RTECS)

Toxic Chemical Release Inventory Files (TRI)

2. *From Other Online Vendors*:

Ovid (databases not available through NLM):

Adis DrugNews—AgeLine—Alcohol and Alcohol Problems Science Database—BioBusiness—BIOSIS Previews—CA Search—CHIROLARS—Combined Health Information Database—Comprehensive Core Medical Library (full text)—Cumulative Index to Nursing and Allied Health—Current Contents—DIOGENES (drug information of FDA)—Drug Information Fulltext—EMBASE—F-D-C Reports—Health and Psychosocial Instruments—Health News Daily—Health Periodicals Database (for laypersons)—International Pharmaceutical Abstracts—Iowa Drug Information Service—Journal Watch (current)—MediConf (medical conferences)—National Epilepsy Library Database—Pharmaceutical and Healthcare Industry News Database—PharmaContacts (pharmaceutical companies)—Pharmaprojects—PNI: Pharmaceutical News Index—PsycINFO—Scientific American Medicine (full text)—SEDBASE (drugs)—SPORT Database (includes sports medicine)

DIALOG (a sampling of databases not available through NLM or Ovid):

American Medical Association Journals Online (full text)—Life Sciences Collection—Mental Health Abstracts—New England Journal of Medicine (full text)—SCISEARCH (*Science Citation Index*)—TSCA Chemical Substances Inventory (toxic substances)—Unlisted Drugs

MEDLINE has been around for a long time and can be accessed from several vendors. The availability of many databases changes. Vendors add databases as well as drop them. In addition, the vendors themselves have been bought out or have taken over other companies. For example, during the summer of 1995, Knight Ridder (parent of DIALOG) announced the acquisition of CARL (parent of UnCover). In 1994 CDP bought BRS and in 1995 renamed itself Ovid. In 1994, also, NLM made its AIDS databases free to search. As well as Paper-

Chase, the NLM is now offering unlimited access to MEDLINE with a fixed annual fee. Physicians Online, Inc., with support from drug companies, offers MEDLINE searching to physicians for free.

Until the 1990s, searchers have accessed online bibliographic databases by means of the telephone line and a modem. It may be faster and cheaper to use the Internet for telecommunications. With your account and password obtained, Telnet to the following:

National Library of Medicine—medlars.nlm.nih.gov

DIALOG Information Services—dialog.com

Ovid—ovid.cdplus.com

PaperChase—pch.bih.harvard.edu

LEXIS-NEXIS—192.73.216.30

OCLC (EPIC)—epic.prod.oclc.org

Also, at some Web sites or Gopher menus on the Internet, subsets of some abstracting and indexing services are searchable for free. Look, for example, at the last six months of CANCERLIT on CancerNet on the NIH Gopher—gopher.nih.gov; this is also accessible via the World Wide Web (WWW)—www.nih.gov. To search a molecular biology subset of MEDLINE for free, use your Web browser to go to http://ncbi.nlm.nih.gov/cgi-bin/medline.

4

Collection Development, Acquisitions, and Cataloging

ORDERING JOURNALS

Searching the literature typically means searching the universe of literature, not just what is in your stacks. Chapter 1 concluded with the factors you consider when deciding which journals to buy for your library. Your next decision concerns ordering. Two routes are available: You can order directly from the publisher, or you can use a serials agent or jobber. Whereas with books libraries expect to buy at a discount, with journals purchasers anticipate extra charges. Serials agents levy a service charge in addition to the price of the journal. To add more injury to the insult, many journals have had two prices: There is a low price for individual subscribers and a high price for libraries. (This issue is independent of the jobber.) There are advantages and disadvantages whether ordering journals directly from the publisher or making purchases through serials jobbers.

Direct to Publishers Advantages (or, Disadvantages of Using a Serials Agent):

1. Restrictive policies of a publisher or agent. Some publishers will not deal with subscription agents and vice versa (e.g., some government document serials). In these cases, there is no choice.
2. Publisher discounts. By ordering several titles from one publisher or society, you may receive a volume discount instead of paying a service charge.

3. No service fee. There is no extra charge when ordering direct. Serials agents charge a percentage of the price of the journal. Their fee may range from 3% to 10%. This adds up to quite a bit of money. If you use agents, evaluate jobbers for their record of service and bargain for favorable rates.
4. No expensive journals' service charges. You may want to order very expensive titles directly. For example, a subscription agent's fee for handling a title like *Brain Research* may be in the hundreds of dollars.

Through Serials Agent Advantages (or, Disadvantages of Ordering Directly to the Publishers):

1. Fewer invoices to take care of. This is an important consideration. Going direct to all the publishers means many invoices and forms and a great deal of paperwork.
2. Avoid publishers' idiosyncrasies. Along with not having to handle all those different invoices, you will not have to understand and comply with all the different ordering procedures.
3. Clout with publishers. For claims of missing issues, the publisher may be more responsive in dealing with a jobber with hundreds of copies at stake than with the problems of your one subscription.
4. Timely information from jobber. Jobbers keep the library informed on title changes, price changes, indexing updates, delayed issues, supplements, and cessations.
5. Automation. Jobber may have an automated system for ordering, checking in, and claiming journals that you will want to use in your library. They may offer online services and CD-ROM products.
6. Foreign journals. You may be able to use the same jobber or a foreign jobber to handle your foreign titles. Often, the choice is made to use a jobber for most of the titles. This service saves the library much time.

The next question to be addressed is which jobber to choose. Comparisons can be made on price and services. What percentage do they charge? What is their record in doing claims and handling supplementary pieces of the publishers, for instance? Are they experienced with biomedical titles and those publishers? Should you look for a vendor that specializes in medical journals and has hospital and medical school libraries among its clients?

SERIALS HANDLING

You have several decisions to make before the journal arrives in the library. For many years, journal issues have been checked in with the use of a Kardex—pull-out files of cards made for this purpose. There is also now the opportunity to do the recordkeeping with a computer. The following is the type of data, examples included, typically held in these records:

Title—*Mechanisms of Ageing and Development*
Publisher—Elsevier

Vendor—Blackwell
ISSN—0047–6374
Purchase Order Number—R023763
Price and Dates Covered by That Price—$1,557/1995
Frequency—21/year
Fund—6805
Library Holdings Information—v.21– , 1983–
Claims—v.75, no.1, July 1994. claimed 10-14-94
Routing Information—Dr. Fain, Box G
Supplements—supplement to v.55: bind in
Binding Information—TP to front; contents and index come in last issue of volume; color: gray
Title Changes—none
Where Shelved—QP86.M47
Binding Record:

Volume	Year	Date Sent	Returned
69–72	1993	2-8-94	2-22-94
73–76	1994	10-24-94	11-8-94

"Routing Information" above brings up a question concerning patron service. For most medical libraries, journals do not circulate. Photocopying an article is usually sufficient for the patron's needs, and the journal can remain in the library for the next person to use. Routine routing of journals to lists of people may be more of an inconvenience to others on the list than it is a convenience for the first person to whom the journal is sent. Small libraries, especially hospital libraries, have used a nice substitute for routing. When the issue arrives, the librarian photocopies the table of contents and sends that to the interested patron. Today there are electronic tables of contents services that can substitute for this paper-based alerting process. A different solution to this is the purchase of duplicate subscriptions. In some cases of heavily used titles, this is desirable. In others, the cost makes the practice prohibitive.

Claiming is another activity noted on the Kardex. Automated services provide an advantage here. You would receive electronic messages when an issue is past due. A big problem with a manual Kardex develops when several issues of a journal are not received. Typically, you will see that an issue has been missed when you check in the one after it. However, if the next one does not come in either, there may not have been a reason to look at that card. Many issues may be missed before it is noticed. Maybe this is a sign that your patrons have not noticed its absence either and are not using it very heavily. In Kardex, keeping on top of claims requires extra diligence.

Journals that you intend to keep more than a year or so need to be bound. If they are not bound, their condition deteriorates through use and sometimes individual issues are lost. The frequency of binding depends on how large a collection you have. There is an alternative to binding if you and your patrons do not mind. Many journals also come in microform. You can receive your current issues in paper but put the collection that you keep in microfiche or microfilm. You will need to acquire adequate machines for reading and printing from the microforms. Remember, as you make your decisions, also to consider the cost of purchase, upkeep, and even replacement. Speaking of machines, functioning photocopying facilities are a must. In most libraries, patrons use self-service photocopiers. Binding interferes with journal use in two ways. Journals sent to the bindery are unavailable to your patrons during that time, and bound volumes are harder to use on photocopy machines than loose issues.

Library staff will need to photocopy journal articles in order to fill interlibrary loan requests. It is not incumbent on you to keep records of the journal copying you do to send out to other libraries. You do, however, need to keep records of the photocopies you receive. Fair use should cover the copying your patrons do. The copying of interlibrary loan requests is allowed by the guidelines that accompany the 1976 revision of the copyright law. Arguments and litigation continue between the publishers and the users of information on copyright law interpretations. Also, the records you have of borrowing (i.e., receipts of photocopies not to be returned) supply valuable use information. If you are requesting copies of articles from the same journal over and over, you should think about subscribing.

SERIALS CATALOGING

In the example of *Mechanisms of Ageing and Development*, that journal was shelved at QP86.M47. This is unusual in two respects. Many medical libraries check in the journals and shelve them in alphabetical order by title instead of call number order. Patrons are very happy with this arrangement. They can go right to the shelves without having to find that library's call number. This usually works well with small collections. The alternative is to catalog the journals and assign classification numbers. In addition to being easy to use, the alphabetical display is less expensive than cataloging and classification, which take staff time and money. There are, however, some advantages to cataloging journals. The classification number keeps journals that are on the same topic near each other on the shelf regardless of the first word of the title:

American Journal of Cardiology

Cardiovascular Research

Journal of Heart Transplantation

Progress in Cardiovascular Diseases

If these "heart" titles are not classified, they are spread apart in the *A*'s, *C*'s, *J*'s, and *P*'s. In addition, among your collection are many serials that have changed titles. If the journal is classified, title changes will not affect the shelving. If the journal is shelved alphabetically, where do you put it, at the current title? at the original title? or at each of the titles, thereby splitting them? Would you consider shelving your current issues in alphabetical order and your bound volumes by call number? The classification number is unusual in another respect. It is a Library of Congress call number. Most medical libraries use the NLM classification, which will be discussed later in the chapter.

TITLE VARIES

In Chapter 1 we saw a bit of the humor of scientists in the *Journal of Irreproducible Results*. The humor of librarians was displayed in a little periodical called *Title Varies*. This small publication made fun of the practices of journals and speculated on the cause of serials librarians' gray hairs. Why do publishers make seemingly trivial changes in titles? Do publishers and editors just have it in for serials librarians? Here is an example from an issue of *Title Varies* (Title Change Hall of Fame 1974).

Bulletin of the Public Health no. 1–46 (1878)

Weekly Abstract of Sanitary Reports (1887)

Public Health Reports (1896)

Public Health Reports absorbed *Journal of Venereal Disease Information, The CDC Bulletin* and *Tuberculosis Control* (1952)

HSMHA Health Reports (1971)

Health Services Reports (1972)

Public Health Reports (1974)

"What May Happen to a Title?" *Serials, Past, Present, and Future* (Brown and Smith 1980) notes many things that may happen to a periodical title. Here are some examples.

—Split: One journal kept the title *Social Science and Medicine* from 1967 to 1977. Over the next few years, it divided into six sections: *Social Science and Medicine. Part A, Medical Sociology, Social Science and Medicine. Part B. Medical Anthropology*, and so on. In 1981 the decision was made to consolidate those parts and return to the original form—one journal called *Social Science and Medicine*.

—Cease publication: *Ulrich's International Periodicals Directory* includes many pages of lists of journals that have stopped publishing.

—Change in format or size: *Bulletin of the Medical Library Association* grew in page size to 8 ½" × 11" in 1989.

—Change titles: *American Academy of Ophthalmology and Otolaryngology: Transactions—Ophthalmology* became *Ophthalmology* in 1978.

—Change numbering: A journal that changes titles may continue its numbering or start again with volume 1. *Federation of American Societies for Experimental Biology. Federation Proceedings* changed title to *FASEB Journal* and started over with a new volume 1.

—Change frequency: *Molecular Microbiology* went from a bimonthly to a monthly two years after it started publication.

Here are a few more happenings. The journal may be suspended for a period of time. The periodical may issue regular or irregular supplements, and these may not include the volume number during that time period. You may choose to keep and bind the supplements with the rest of the journal, or you may catalog each separately to be its own monograph. Another thing can happen to a journal title that you order and pay for: It may never arrive. Serials librarians will be happy to tell you stories including the mysteries of the mail.

BIBLIOGRAPHIC TOOLS FOR JOURNALS

Some tools useful for obtaining bibliographic and ordering information about journals are listed below. For brand-new or forthcoming titles, the publishers' announcements may be the only information available.

Ulrich's International Periodicals Directory

Serials Directory

Standard Periodical Directory

Union List of Serials (1950)

New Serial Titles (1950–)

Vendor tools such as: Faxon's *Librarians' Guide to Serials* and EBSCO's *Librarians' Handbook*

Lists of serials included in abstracting and indexing services; examples include *List of Journals Indexed in Index Medicus, Serial Sources for the BIOSIS Previews Database, Chemical Abstracts Service Source Index.*

Regional union lists such as *Union Catalog of Medical Periodicals* (UCMP)

Computer databases, including OCLC (Online Computers Library Center), RLIN (Research Libraries Information Network, Research Libraries Group), SERLINE (SERials onLINE, an NLM database)

ELECTRONIC JOURNAL

We have traveled through the entire process of (1) viewing the nature and roles of journals; (2) evaluating needs and selecting journals; (3) searching the journal literature for articles on specific subjects; (4) budgeting for journals and deciding on the appropriate ways to acquire them; (5) checking in the serials, keeping track of them, routing them, binding them, and so on. This is the traditional path. The journal system has served several useful functions, as we have seen, but it has also attracted many complaints. The capability for widespread transmission of electronic text is here, and electronic journals already exist. Given the time delay and expense of paper production, will the traditional journal last?

Kassirer and Angell (1995) noted their concerns with the lack of quality control of information on the Internet. Let us propose here that those functions of peer review and gatekeeping can be moved successfully to the electronic journal. What, then, are the prospects for the paper journals and the electronic journals? Will electronic journals be available by individual article, by whole journal issue, by annual subscription, or by all of these? Will they be less expensive or more expensive than paper journals? Will electronic journals really be just the same as the paper ones but presented by different means? Will the technology change the essence of the product? Will the illustrations be better? Will sound be added? Will the journal be multimedia? If journals are available article by article, and that is how they are purchased, will students have as much access to them as they have today? More? Less? What will happen to sciences libraries if article-by-article access comes to dominate journal transmission? Document delivery is now popular among many individuals and libraries. Will there be a need for health sciences libraries? Will our traditional patrons go directly to the source and see us as irrelevant caretakers of the older, pre-electronic information?

The first fully planned, impressively sponsored, and prominently edited electronic journal was the *Online Journal of Current Clinical Trials* (OJCCT). Dissemination of findings from clinical trials certainly demands timeliness and is a fitting role for an electronic journal. The OJCCT was announced to the medical community and the library community well in advance of its initial publication. There was much anticipation and, in the library community, at least, excitement. The publishers were the American Association for the Advancement of Science (AAAS) and OCLC, organizations of great weight in science and librarianship respectively. The editor was Edward J. Huth, former editor of *Annals of Internal Medicine*. A new piece of software, Guidon, was developed for use with this journal. Peer review for the articles was accomplished in the traditional way. The subscription was $100 per year—certainly modest by biomedical journal standards. The method of distribution was the difference. Subscribers logged in via the Internet or phone lines or dedicated OCLC lines and then entered their authorization password. They may or may not have used the special software. Later, in 1992, IM began to index the OJCCT. The problem was that the manuscripts submitted to OJCCT were few. Although OJCCT was backed by formidable organizations and had all the makings of a prominent journal, not many authors submitted their papers to it. The electronic journal was not embraced as swiftly as expected. Despite its prestigious pedigree, OJCCT did not find immediate success. Innovations in electronic publishing nonetheless continue (Hickey 1995). Many publishers do sell their journals on CD-ROM as well as in paper (e.g., *Annals of Internal Medicine, JAMA,* and *New England Journal of Medicine*). Many electronic newsletters and some journals can be searched now without a personal subscription fee on the Internet.

JOURNALS VERSUS MONOGRAPHIC SERIALS

The terms "books" and "journals" seem clear and distinct. "Journal" does sound more lofty than "magazine." The publications referred to here may be called journals, periodicals, serials, or magazines. A unifying characteristic is that there is no planned end in sight. The publisher intends to produce the publication into the indefinite future. Another type of publication that may or may not have a planned ending is the monographic serial. The monographic serial differs from the monographic set; a "set" indicates that an ending volume is planned. The difference between a journal and a monographic series is not as obvious. Each number (i.e., issue) of a monographic series is usually a book that can stand on its own. It is a monograph. However, in a series, the publisher links the individual numbers together. A library can order a series with a subscription or by purchasing individual pieces as they come out. An example of a monographic series is *Progress in Clinical and Biological Research.* Here are titles of a few volumes within that series: *Drug and Chemical Risks to the Fetus and Newborn; Genetics of Kidney Disorders*; and *Tumor Viruses*. Each title is on a completely different topic and can stand on its own.

Monographic series may be thought of as a convenience to the library. You may want to get all the volumes and can order a subscription, as you would with ordinary journals. You may instead consider this linking of disparate titles as an underhanded scheme by the publisher to sell more books. Once the volumes come into the library, you may also choose how you will handle them—as a single journal title or as separately cataloged books. On the one hand, patrons will be able to identify additional books on the subject they are seeking if you catalog them individually. On the other hand, patrons see the citations to *Progress in Clinical and Biological Research* as journal articles within a serial title in IM. Monographic series may be numbered or unnumbered. In either case, you need to recognize them as different from your primary journals, and you must handle them as appropriate to your patrons' needs.

BOOKS: COLLECTION DEVELOPMENT

What about books? Where do books fit in? An important function of journals is to communicate the recent research findings, and the articles usually presume that the reader has a certain familiarity with the topic. Articles do not typically supply well-organized and broad pictures of a field. Their focus is very narrow. It would be difficult for a person new to the subject area to jump directly into the journal literature. Books provide the systematic background for the scientific literature, as they would in any discipline. The problem with books is that they are out of date before they are published. Although this is true of other disciplines, even health sciences librarianship, with medicine this fact is pointed out more often. The previous two chapters discussed how to link up a person's specific need with answers found in the literature of the field. Health sciences librarianship places a heavy emphasis on reference service with a secondary status for collection development. We have routinely looked beyond our own holdings since the development of an efficient interlibrary loan network in the 1960s. In this sense we have been ahead of other types of libraries. In a small medical library, we have always taken this position: emphasis on access instead of emphasis on ownership.

SELECTION

What books will you be purchasing for your library? The demand for scientific currency does make it easier. Unless your collection is atypical of a health sciences library and emphasizes historical material, you will be able to concentrate on the current literature. This is the key factor. Taking into account the vagaries of the publishing industry and the short time books may be in print, new books are still relatively easy to acquire. You will not need to spend much time and effort tracking down rare books or dealing with out-of-print dealers. You will not have to do a great deal of retrospective selection to build up a collection on a topic new to your institution. Also, most of our patrons do not have proficiencies in languages beyond English. That situation and the fact that English is the dominant language in medicine means that we will not usually need to purchase foreign-language materials. English-language materials are certainly published within many countries, but our transactions with foreign publishers will be fewer than for our colleagues in the humanities libraries. The need for current information also means that the books must be obtained quickly. If we are to believe that the books are out of date when published, the least we can do is to get them into the hands of the patrons as quickly as possible.

Since a medical library is a special library, to a greater or lesser extent the collection focuses on relatively few subjects. The needs of a particular institution dictate what is to be bought, of course. That may be the point to remember throughout the succeeding discussions of core lists, approval plans, and so on. For example, if you are the librarian at a psychiatric hospital, your collection probably focuses on psychiatry and psychology and does not have a great deal on gastroenterology or cancer medicine. If your library is serving a biomedical research institution that has as its mission the investigation of lung physiology and lung diseases, those topics dictate what you need to purchase. If your library serves a medical school, a dental school, a veterinary medical school, a nursing school, a pharmacy school, an allied health school, and a teaching hospital, the collection will be very broad within the health sciences.

How much of what you need should you buy? "Access as opposed to ownership" is a nice idea and a compelling ideology in the face of our budgets. As more and more materials are produced and available in electronic form, it is an idea whose time will come. Now, however, it is fine for items that are needed occasionally. Until we move somewhat further along to our virtual library, publications and sources that are continuously used need to be on hand. What percentage of materials within your core topics will you be able to buy? Can you ever be comprehensive? It may be possible. The library supporting research in lung physiology and disease, for example, may find that the universe of publications relating specifically to the lung and respiratory system may be small enough to attempt to cover it exhaustively. It would still be difficult to get all the journal articles in the field because the relevant literature would be scattered over many journals. The Bradford Distribution (see Chapter 1) helps somewhat. Medical libraries have done very well in their resource sharing of the journal literature, but books have not fit into the system as neatly. Locator tools did not develop as quickly for books as for journals. However, now that has changed with Internet access to other libraries' online catalogs and union lists (e.g., OCLC). In deciding what you needed to buy, you would also have checked whether other biomedical libraries were situated near you and if they were open to your clientele. Perhaps that question loses some significance with the advent of fax machines and other sophisticated telecommunications devices, but books are usually sent the old-fashioned way. It is easy to envision the technological feasibility of electronic journals, too. What about a future for electronic books or the development of optical scanning of text? Regardless of the type of your library and the state of the art of technology and your sharing arrangements, you need to make clear your own collecting intentions. You can do this in your collection development policy.

COLLECTION DEVELOPMENT POLICY

It may be that you have been running your library for years and that you know all your patrons and understand their information needs. You may also have a firm grip on the literature and confidently and wisely handle your selection activities. However, even then it will be useful to have a document, a written collection development policy. Your patrons and administrators need to be able to see the plan you have, to know what to expect, and to understand how you, the librarian, are endeavoring to serve the institution. Your collecting follows the direction you have set, and the document will make it clear to others. Also, accrediting agencies may require a library to have a policies and procedures manual (see Chapter 7 on hospital librarianship). The collection development policy is an important part of the manual and should cover the following.

1. *Authority.* The collection development policy should assign the authority for the collection. Who is responsible for the collection? In a one-person hospital library, only one person seems to have the responsibility. Yet it may not be that clear-cut. Most hospitals as well as other institutions have a library committee. The library committee is useful in setting policies and goals for the library, and its members may be very helpful as advocates of the library to the administration of the parent organization. Members of the library committee may also involve themselves directly in purchasing decisions. This is frequently the case in selecting expensive journals. If several of the medical departments are represented,

the committee may be a suitable forum for discussing and ranking the many new journals under consideration. The collection development policy should spell out the responsibilities and roles of the librarian and the library committee. At the same time, the librarian needs to ensure that the patrons' needs are addressed. In any case, the composition of the library committee should be covered in the policy. In larger libraries, collection decisions are often dispersed among several librarians. A university medical library may divide the subject areas among the reference librarians.

2. *Direction and Depth.* The collection development policy spells out the direction in which the collection is going. The goals and purposes of the larger institution are reflected in the policy, which delineates the subjects to be covered and the depth to which each subject should be collected. These matters may be addressed in a narrative form and with charts. Categories of subjects may be listed by their range of classification numbers in your library. Each call number group may then be given a ranking. The rankings originated by the ALA are widely used and convenient for larger libraries. There are five ALA levels:

Comprehensive—trying to be exhaustive; attempting to get everything you identify for a defined subject area.

Research—getting material necessary to support doctoral-level research programs. This involves extensive collecting.

Study—collecting up to, but not including, doctoral-level research projects.

Basic—much more selective; supplying representative items for disciplines.

Minimal—rarely selecting in a subject area that is out of the scope for your library.

Here is a sample entry for a collection development policy using these ALA levels.

WL 1–225	Anatomy, Physiology, Neurochemistry	S	R for Blood-Brain Barrier
WL 300–405	Central Nervous System	S	R for Epilepsy
WL 500–544	Peripheral Nerves	R	
WL 600–610	Autonomic Nervous System	S	
WL 700–710	Sense Organs	B	

Health sciences libraries have widely varying collections and very different collection development policies. The *Collection Development Manual of the National Library of Medicine* describes selection activities of one of the national libraries. For areas within the scope of the library's mission, many of the subjects are to be collected comprehensively. However, a number of areas of interest to NLM are not collected in an all-encompassing fashion. For instance, veterinary medicine is collected at the research level. NLM also recognized that another national library, the National Agricultural Library, will be collecting heavily in veterinary medicine. Popular works on medicine, those written at the lay level, are collected more thoroughly by the Library of Congress than by NLM. The third edition of NLM's collection policy—initially available over the Internet—came out in 1993. Here is its guidance to selectors for two selected subjects: ''Cardiology'' and ''Health Services Research''

CARDIOLOGY
Definition: The branch of medicine concerned with the heart and cardiovascular system.
(National Library of Medicine 1993b, 20)
HEALTH SERVICES RESEARCH
Definition: The scientific study of the effect of health care delivery and management on health care access, quality, and cost.
Includes:

- Analysis of health care costs, insurance, utilization, availability, and accessibility
- Assessment of health status, health care need and demand
- Assessment of health care technology and effectiveness of quality assurance techniques
- Assessment of patient and health outcomes
- Assessment of the effectiveness of health education and patient instruction
- Development of clinical practice guidelines and health standards, and analysis of their effectiveness
- Evaluation of the impact of health care and administrative management strategies on health care delivery
- Health planning and forecasting

Note: Health services research uses statistical and epidemiological techniques to plan, assess, and evaluate the effect or impact of various factors on health outcomes and effective health care delivery. Health services research also utilizes a variety of social and behavioral research techniques.

See also: EPIDEMIOLOGY
HEALTH CARE TECHNOLOGY
HEALTH ECONOMICS
HEALTH SERVICES
MEDICAL SOCIOLOGY
(National Library of Medicine 1993b, 29)

The collection development policy briefly notes an established medical specialty (CARDIOLOGY), but a new area of research and practice (HEALTH SERVICES RESEARCH) includes details of its scope and explanations of what it is. Put directions and reminders in your collection development policy to make it a useful working document for your selection of materials.

3. *Types of Material.* The types of material to be purchased need to be understood and specified (e.g., textbooks, treatises, workbooks). A medical textbook, for instance, is not like an introductory text for a subject. Practitioners

see these medical books as codifications of state-of-the-art information and use them in their everyday treatment of patients. Consider this sampling of questions to address. Will you be buying introductory material? Will you keep older editions? Will you be getting books that include computer disks and other media? Do you have the equipment to handle the disks? Are you collecting handbooks, laboratory manuals, loose-leaf services, paperbound books, or programmed texts? Do you want books with a scholarly approach and explanations of theory or ones with an applied orientation? For subjects within your institution's interests, do you want business, legal, or ethical aspects? Are you willing to obtain foreign-language material? Do you need to look for translations?

How might you handle published symposia proceedings? There are several potential problems with these publications. They are often characterized as being variable in quality. Because most of them have many contributors, some sections of a publication may be valuable and well written, whereas other papers are incomplete and unedited. The information in some may be timely characterizations of what is happening in a field and be the only source available on a topic. Others may contain fragmentary notes on subjects or have publication dates years after the date of the meeting. Some may be poorly written and poorly produced. They may be expensive. Many of the papers may already have appeared or may soon appear as edited articles in journals. Libraries single out these publications for direction in the policy because of their abundance, cost, and quality.

4. *Collection Level.* You know what subject areas to collect. However, you also need to tailor the subject collections to the level of the patrons. Your institution may be involved in teaching, research, and clinical care. It may have a pharmacy internship program, cancer research projects, medical students on rotation in the hospital, and heart surgery specialists. A topic can be covered by numerous books at many levels for different audiences. Let's assume, for example, that research on aphasia—disorders in the use, understanding, or production of language—is being done at your institution. You collect monographs and journals in the neurosciences and psychology to support this area. Are you buying material for patient care, nursing, social work, or even lay literature in addition to publications for the neurologists, neurosurgeons, and neuropsychologists? Are you getting materials from the National Head Injury Foundation for the use of patients and their families? You may want to buy different books on the same topic at different levels, or you may not. Your purchasing choices depend on the audiences you serve.

5. *Budget.* The prices of materials are factors in many decisions. For instance, how much of your budget can be allocated for periodicals and still leave enough money for books? Journal prices have been rising faster than the price of other materials in your library; these, in turn, have been rising faster than the general rate of inflation. If you are going to be able to buy any books at all, you will need either to put a leash on your serials budget or to increase the library's

share of the budget pie. Whatever the budget level, you must think about what percentage should go to serials and what percentage should be spent on books. There have been studies on this topic. Burdick, Butler, and Sullivan (1993) examined citation practices in medical books and journals. They found that 88% of the references were to serials, with 12% for books. A citation record that can be counted on to reflect proportional use may be a helpful guide for relative spending. In your policy, mention the inflation factor as well as trends in biomedical book publishing. Do books follow that path of specialization the way serials do? Many books are published on very narrow topics, and this limits the potential audience for them. How many of these very specialized monographs can you justify buying? The pricing practices of the publishers of journals have caused problems for libraries. What about the prices of medical books? The Brandon list (addressed later in the chapter) of 610 medical books gives an average price of $110.95 in 1995 (Brandon and Hill 1995). Many of the medical texts are expensive, even allowing that they often have more than one volume (e.g., *Heart Disease: A Textbook of Cardiovascular Medicine*, two-volume set at $131.75; *Campbell's Operative Orthopaedics*, five-volume set at $450). For heavily demanded items, can you afford to purchase duplicates? Sometimes books are published that are cumulations of papers previously published elsewhere. Do you want to avoid this duplication or do you want the collections of classic articles for the convenience of your patrons? What are your policies and procedures for audiovisuals? software programs? electronic products? Are there specific procedures in place for selecting very expensive books or for starting journal subscriptions? What happens when the needs of your patrons, reflected in the range and depth set forward in your collecting policy, meet the realities of your budget? What do you do when you cannot afford what you need to buy? Do you specify what amount of the budget is to go to each of the medical specialties or subjects (e.g., pediatrics, molecular biology, cardiology)? Theoretically, gifts may be a form of budget relief. Do you have a policy on gifts? Unfortunately, gifts may be runs of old medical journals that are owned by everybody or outdated medical texts.

6. *History*. What is the history of the collection? What are its strengths? Is your institution continuing work in its traditional areas? Is there an obligation to continue to collect in those strong areas of the collection? This is not a rhetorical question. If, indeed, the hospital is no longer involved with delivering babies or if the funding for research in diabetes has been eliminated, the library need not and often cannot afford to purchase materials at former levels in those subjects. In some instances, resource-sharing agreements may encourage you to continue collecting as part of reciprocal agreements.

7. *Approval Plans*. The role of gathering plans, discussed later in the chapter, should be addressed in the collection development policy.

8. *Collections for Support Services*. What about those areas not directly within the main missions of your institution—those areas that are not clinical, research, or teaching? What about information and materials for support services (e.g., hospital administration)? These need the services of the library, too.

9. *Outside Users.* Are there noninstitutional users of the library? Public librarians? Outside researchers? Patients? The public with consumer health questions? The health literature designed for the consumer differs from the literature for the health care professionals. You may not traditionally have collected such literature, but your organization may now want to become involved in the growing consumer wellness movement.

10. *Growth of the Literature.* The collection development policy should also acknowledge the growth of the biomedical literature both for the purpose of cost and for the problem of space limitations that you will likely have. Can part of your collection be moved to a remote facility? Are the conversions of back runs of journals to microforms and the use of electronic products viable options for the library?

11. *Collection Evaluation and Weeding.* Weeding is the other side of selection. One part of the decisions on what to weed will again be dictated by the mission of your institution. If you are supporting mainly clinical care, you may want to get rid of older, superseded editions. Some new editions do not incorporate all still-valid material from the older editions. If your collection supports research in a field, it will be necessary to keep more of the older material. Do you have a plan in place for ongoing reviews of the adequacy of your collection? Institutions often take up new objectives, and individuals' needs do not stay the same year after year. You need to interview new staff to find out their specialties and information needs. Also, do periodic surveys of all users' needs to keep the collection and your services up-to-date for them.

12. *Resource Sharing.* Resource sharing as a way to meet service needs should be explained. The arrangements with other organizations and libraries need to be spelled out in your policy. Interlibrary loan and document delivery take care of part of the issue. What about cooperative purchasing arrangements with other libraries? You might consider a formal arrangement that recognizes the strengths of the various libraries in your consortium and assigns collection-building responsibilities among them. This applies to cancellations of journal subscriptions, too. Can you work out an agreement with other institutions so that all the libraries do not cancel the same journals? More and more tools are becoming available to the end user (e.g., CD-ROM and remote databases). This stimulates the demand for articles, books, documents, and so on. With this increased demand, can you really justify the reduced role of ownership that we are either committed to or resigned to? Also, your smaller collection removes opportunities for browsing. Do electronic alerting services adequately replace the loss? Although you may not be able to supply satisfactory answers to all these questions, you certainly need to consider these issues.

SOURCES OF INFORMATION ABOUT NEW BOOKS

Now that the policy is in place, how do you go about selecting the materials? Where can you locate information about new books—those just published or about to be published?

1. *Publishers' Flyers and Catalogs*. If the order of the entries in this listing were based on volume, this certainly would be the number one source. You will receive a lot of notices from the publishers about the availability of new books. The flyers give detailed information, tables of contents, and favorable comments. In addition, representatives of publishers sometimes telephone you or visit you in the library.

2. *Vendors' Flyers and Catalogs*. Book vendors will do the same thing as publishers. The communications from them may be in the traditional paper catalogs or through their online systems. They will also inevitably supply you with multiple copies of their offerings.

3. *Library Patrons' Requests*. Library patrons also receive flyers and catalogs from publishers. They go to medical meetings of their specialty, where they encounter the publishers, and then they find themselves on the publisher's mailing lists. Your patrons are valuable sources for book recommendations about the quality of the books and how they may be relevant to their work. It is your responsibility, however, to see that everyone's information needs are met. Inevitably, some people are outspoken about their needs. This means that you will not be able to rely solely on the requests from your patrons for the selection of materials.

4. *CATLINE and Locator*. One of the NLM databases is CATLINE. This is NLM's online catalog. Because NLM is the world's largest library devoted to a single subject, medicine, it is a good source for bibliographic information on books. Until recently CATLINE was available mainly in the same way all the other databases on the MEDLARS system are, namely, by online connection and subsequent charges. In 1993 NLM Locator became available on the Internet. Locator includes CATLINE, AVLINE for audiovisuals, and SERLINE for information on journal titles. Now that you can search these databases without a password and without charges, two paper publications have been discontinued: *Current Catalog Proof Sheets* and *Current Catalog*. The former was a weekly listing of new books in the health sciences; the latter was a quarterly and annual cumulation. The former ended in 1992 and the latter in 1993. (The *National Library of Medicine Audiovisuals Catalog* also was discontinued in 1993.) This is an indication of the direction of information sources: first, print; then the simultaneous production of print and computer; and finally, computer only.

5. *Interlibrary Loan Records*. For publications that are not brand new, interlibrary loan records may tell you what your patrons want that you do not own. This will be particularly appropriate for journal subscriptions.

6. *Book Advertisements in Medical Journals*. This is another source of information for you and for your patrons. Like publisher and vendor announcements, these should offer timely information.

With the possible exception of your patrons' requests, these sources do not give relatively unbiased evaluations of the books. Advertisements may supply full descriptions but could not be considered impartial. Where do you go to get more information about a book—more than merely, say, the bibliographic information? Just as you would with other fields, find a book review.

BOOK REVIEWS

The main problem with book reviews has been tardiness. It takes so much time for the review of the book to be published that the review is not useful in the selection decision. We usually need to acquire the book when it is released if we are going to get it at all. Timely reviews would certainly help. Actually, some medical journals often include reviews of recently published books. The weekly, general interest, and widely read medical journals noted in Chapter 1 are sources to start with (i.e., *JAMA*, *Lancet*, and the *New England Journal of Medicine*).

If you had come across a citation or an advertisement for a book and wanted to find a review, where would you go? You could go to one of the above to scan the latest issues. If the book is a little older, you could go to an annual index of journals to look at the list of books reviewed. You might check specialized medical journals that have reviews covering their specialty. This seems a bit haphazard and time consuming. There is no equivalent to the *Book Review Digest* or the *Book Review Index* for the fields of interest to us. In the early 1980s the Institute for Scientific Information published the *Index to Book Reviews in the Sciences*. This helpfully supplied an index to reviews written in the journals that it indexed, and many medical journals were included. Perhaps libraries found the price too high or the reviews too late to help. This publication lasted only a few years. There was a publication for reviews of reference books that included biomedicine, *Science and Technology Annual Reference Review*. It covered only reference materials and lasted from 1988 to 1991. Although MEDLINE does not index book reviews, you might search some databases that do (e.g., *Academic Index* or *Books in Print Plus*). The Association of College and Research Libraries publishes *Choice*. Also available in cards, these are book reviews in all fields that have particular relevance for academic libraries. Again comes the question of timeliness. This problem was addressed in 1993 with the publication of *Doody's Health Sciences Book Review Journal*. With your subscription, in 1995 it became searchable via the Internet.

Is waiting for a book review usually out of the question? Would book reviews still be of use to librarians even several months after publication? Truelson (1976) and Almagro (1984) maintained that there is a time for book reviews. That time is when budgets are tight. With less money to spend, it may be reasonable to wait to make sure that the books in question are the most suitable for your collection. Almagro listed the journals in each medical specialty that have regular book review sections. For example, the section on neurology lists fifteen journals, including *Brain; Journal of Neurology, Neurosurgery, and Psychiatry;* and *Trends in Neurosciences*. The article is several years old, but that does not matter. You can use this idea by finding the journals with book reviews in your fields and scan them regularly. Almagro also makes a plea to the journal editors and reviewers to act more speedily. Some databases, although not MEDLINE, index book reviews (Goddard 1993).

How valuable is the book review? You read reviews, and they all seem positive. Kroenke (1986) found that impression to be largely true. Favorable reviews in medical journals are common, he found: favorable, 88.5 percent; unfavorable, 11.5 percent. That being the case, why would they be worth waiting for? What explains the lopsided figures? Perhaps only the better books are selected for reviewing? Many books are received but few are chosen for review. Perhaps reviewers strain to say something positive about any book. Perhaps reviewers are too timid to write a negative review, fearing either professional repercussions or personal antagonism. Remember, beyond examining a book's quality, a reviewer can identify the appropriate audiences for a book, and that will be useful to us.

Small and large libraries use reviews differently. Small hospital libraries do not buy many books per year. They must be quite selective, and reviews can help. At the other extreme is NLM. "It is impractical for NLM to give consideration to estimates of quality in acquiring printed literature for the collection" (National Library of Medicine 1985, 1). In other words, if the subject matter fits the scope of the collection, NLM wants to acquire it. The library does not try to be comprehensive in every subject. Also, NLM looks at quality considerations for nonprint materials.

CORE LISTS

Most medical specialties recognize particular books as authorities for that field. How did the books get to be authorities? These texts are used by students in medical school. After those students become physicians, they rely on the texts they are familiar with—their schoolbooks—in their clinical care decisions. New editions come out frequently. Many of the original authors have long since died, but often their names are carried on in the titles. *Harrison's Principles of Internal Medicine; Goodman and Gilman's Pharmacological Basis of Therapeutics; Williams Obstetrics;* and *Zinsser Microbiology* are a few of these. Core lists of these authoritative works are widely disseminated and used. They are compiled by librarians and physicians and published in library journals, medical journals, and nursing journals. One is updated and published every other year in the *Bulletin of the Medical Library Association*'s "Selected List of Books and Journals for the Small Medical Library" (Brandon and Hill 1995). Alfred N. Brandon and Dorothy R. Hill are the librarian authors of this widely known "Brandon list"—also called Brandon-Hill. Composed of books and journals, the list has a subset of materials designated as initial purchases for the very small medical library. The books are grouped (e.g., anatomy, biochemistry, cardiovascular system). The authors of this list do not maintain that it is necessary to buy all the books in a given category. Yet it is good to understand that these are books that your clientele will often request.

Another well-used list, "A Library for Internists," is published in the *Annals of Internal Medicine* every third year and has as its author and compiler a physician (Mazza 1994). Subtitled "Recommendations from the American College of Physicians," this list formerly included journals. Each book's citation is accompanied by a brief annotation. The Brandon list has the bibliographic data but no annotation. Mazza, like Brandon, notes that one need not buy all the titles in each subject group.

Brandon and Hill compile lists of books and journals for other areas of the health sciences, too. Every other year "Selected List of Nursing Books and Journals" (Brandon and Hill 1994a) is published in a nursing journal. Another list from these two librarians is "Selected List of Books and Journals in Allied Health Sciences" (Brandon and Hill 1994b) and is found in the *Bulletin of the Medical Library Association*. In a way, this list may be the most helpful of all for the health sciences librarian. Support in health sciences libraries for allied health may often not be up to the more traditional disciplines of medicine and nursing. (A case in point: The book in hand has certainly emphasized "medical" information so far.) The authors' "focus has been directed primarily to the twenty-eight educational programs accredited by the Committee on Allied Health Education and Accreditation (CAHEA) of the American Medical Association, plus physical therapy, dental allied health, medical secretarial, nutrition, and speech pathology/audiology programs" (Brandon and Hill 1994a: 247). As with the medical list, these latter two have subsets for initial purchases.

JUDGING BOOKS FOR SELECTION

How might you view these and other core lists? They may be useful to you in a few ways. Like reviews, they may be too late. However, many of these books are new editions of ones that have been around for a long time. You will be alert for an announcement of a new edition. Although there is no guarantee that the succeeding edition will be as well done as the last one you bought, the odds are good. The needs of your clientele may be met by a portion of the titles on the core lists, so you should adapt these lists to your situation.

You also need to order books that are not on lists. How do you decide what to buy? You must understand the subject needs of your institution. Faced with the books, how can you judge quality? The majority of the publications you purchase are of a very specialized nature. You are probably not an authority in these fields. Even if you were an authority in some areas, you are not likely to be an authority in all. It will therefore be difficult for you to make a quality judgment based on a subject analysis of the content. One factor to consider is the publisher. You will become expert as you get to know the major medical publishers. There will be publishers who regularly issue quality material of interest for your institution. Below is a listing of publishers with the numbers of books each had on earlier medical (Brandon and Hill 1993), nursing (Brandon and Hill 1992b), and allied health (Brandon and Hill 1992a) lists compiled by Brandon and Hill. A few of the books appear on more than one list, so there is some duplication. The publishers are listed if they had more than one book on any one of the three lists. This is intended to show some of the important publishers in health care and is not the universe that you will deal with. Basic health sciences books are not represented here. Another reminder: since take-overs and mergers happen regularly among publishers, some names of publishers listed here will change.

Publisher	Medical	Nursing	Allied Health
Addison Wesley Nursing	2	12	
American Hospital Association	2		
American Medical Association	5		2
American Psychiatric Press	8		
American Society for Microbiology	2		1
Appleton & Lange	45	32	21
Aspen	11	25	20
Benjamin Cummings		1	4
Blackwell	5		
Brady			12
Churchill Livingstone	18		15
Davis	2	18	39
Delmar	2	7	13
Elsevier	2		1
Health Administration Press	2		
Johns Hopkins	3		
Jones and Bartlett	4	16	1
Lea & Febiger	32		23
Lippincott	67	38	30
Little, Brown	45		16
McGraw-Hill	25	2	
Macmillan	1		2
Medical Economics Data	2		
Medical Examinations Publishing Co			2
Merck	3		
Mosby Year Book	92	108	86
National Academy Press	2		2
Oxford University Press	9		

Plenum	2		
Prentice Hall	1		6
Raven	10		4
Saunders	121	37	39
Slack			6
Springer Publishing Co.	1	12	
Springer-Verlag	2		2
Springhouse Corp.	1	10	1
Thomas	1		6
Thieme	1		2
Wiley-Liss	2		
Williams & Wilkins	44	6	26
Totals (all publishers)	606	325	396

For comparison, here are the numbers for the most prolific publishers on the latest medical list (Brandon and Hill 1995).

Saunders	113
Mosby	96
Williams & Wilkins	62
Little, Brown	57
Lippincott	55
Appleton & Lange	48
McGraw-Hill	33
Churchill Livingstone	15

You will be dealing with some other medical publishers also: Academic Press, Allyn & Bacon, American Academy of Orthopaedic Surgeons, American Academy of Pediatrics, American Board of Medical Specialties, American Dental Association, American Nurses Association, American Pharmacy Association, American Psychological Association, American Public Health Association, Bailliere Tindall, Basic Books, Butterworths, Cambridge, Charles Press, CRC Press, Dekker, Facts & Comparisons, Freeman, Grune & Stratton, HarperCollins, Harvard University, Hemisphere, Igaku-Shoin, IRL Press, Joint Commission on Accreditation of Healthcare Organizations, Jossey-Bass, Karger, Kluwer, Lexington, Macmillan, MIT Press, National League for Nursing, Parthenon, Pergamon, Physicans Desk Reference, Praeger, Quality Medical Publishing, Taylor & Francis, U.S. Pharmacopeia, University of Chicago Press, Urban & Schwarzenberg, Van Nostrand, Wadsworth, West Publishing, and Yale University Press.

For small libraries, the judgment of quality is even more important because few books are bought. The other end of the spectrum is the NLM with its comprehensive approach to collecting. Another way to assign a quality rating may be on the basis of the author. Over time you will become familiar with many authors in the medical field. Another source of help can come from the patrons using the materials. Consulting the physicians or nurses or researchers about some of the books that you are unsure of has a bonus, too. A favorable recommendation alerts them to the book, so they will likely use it when it comes in.

APPROVAL PLANS

For larger libraries, a gathering or approval plan may be useful. An approval plan works like this. The library contracts with one or more jobbers that offer approval plans. The library discusses the subjects that it collects and the extent to which they are collected. In essence, the vendor needs to understand, in detail, the library's collection development policy. The vendor receives books continuously from publishers. When a book comes in that matches your library's profile, the book is sent to you. The great advantage of this is the timeliness. You do not have to wait to find out about the book and then go through the procedures to order it. With a good approval plan and vendor, the needed books should be in your hands more quickly. If you see that the book does not happen to meet your specifications, send it back. Books are sent on approval. However, neither you nor the vendor wants to have a lot of books sent back. If you find that you are returning a large percentage of the books, you should either go over your profile again with the vendor or consider another vendor. With an approval plan, you may get an extra discount for arranging this volume business.

What are the disadvantages? It may be difficult to set up an approval plan that works well for you. You may need to do the book selecting yourself. Many of the books you receive may not be appropriate. Of course, there may be many books you should be getting but are not. If you have to monitor the book announcements to protect yourself from not missing books as you did before the approval plan, your approval plan is not doing much for you. There may a negative economic effect, too. You may be reluctant to return the books you would not have otherwise ordered, saying to yourself, "Well, this will round out the collection." Do you really have the money to satisfy peripheral interests? Some dealers specialize in medical books. Having their expertise in place before they start on your order will be helpful. Does the vendor include the publishers you use? Can purchasing procedures be worked out between the vendor and your purchasing department to ensure a smoothly running system? For the returns, does the vendor pay the postage? Instead of sending the books, can the vendor supply announcements for items that may be peripheral in your library's profile? This can alert you, for example, to the symposium proceeding you do want to buy. Does reliance on an approval plan mean you will be getting the same books from the same publishers that every other library gets? Does this shortchange the particular needs of your clientele?

Related to approval plans are standing orders and continuation orders of series. Your library may find it convenient to make arrangements with a publisher to receive books automatically. One difference is that you are getting these books through firm orders. This is different from an approval plan and the books are not to be sent back.

ORDERING PROCEDURES

Verify book information before ordering. The sources noted earlier for finding information about new books can be use here, as well. In addition, use the bibliographic utilities, OCLC and RLIN, and the online catalogs of other libraries. After determining the bibliographic details, find out if the book you want is in print. Beyond the regular *Books in Print* is *Medical and Health Care Books and Serials in Print*. For ordering, decide whether the library is going directly to the publisher, using a book jobber, or relying on standing orders and approval plans. You should be able to get a discount on your book orders, unlike journal orders. Also take the opportunity to use online ordering through a number of vendors. Book-ordering procedures are the same for health sciences libraries as for any other type. For insight into the relationships among libraries, publishers, and vendors, see an ALA book on acquisitions (Schmidt 1990).

One more word about the ordering procedures. They may not be up to you. Your institution may have ordering methods that may or may not work well with books. Some institutions require the contract sent out to bid. Your organization may participate in statewide contracts. There are also arrangements wherein the ordering for the individual libraries of a group is consolidated and done by the head office (e.g., Veterans Administration hospitals).

DYNAMIC BOOKS

Books do not now have to be viewed as static publications. They can become "dynamic" a number of ways. Publications-on-demand are available at some bookstores that serve college campuses, the professors, and their students. With the computerized production of books, bookstores are downloading parts of different books to create "new" books for the needs of specific college courses. This offshoot of traditional publishing must be done under the appropriate authority and by arrangement with and royalty payments to the original publishers. For many years Prentice Hall and the Bureau of National Affairs produced looseleaf services to keep people up to date on laws and regulations. Every week or month or quarter replacement pages would arrive for the publication. *Scientific American Medicine* has been published with the same idea. Instead of issuing a whole new edition in two or three years, updates are sent throughout the year. *Consult*, the CD-ROM version of *Scientific American Medicine*, provides an updated, replacement disk every three months. With the CD-ROM version, the whole book is searchable, so that the reader can find each occurrence of every word in the book. There is also the potential to incorporate sound and moving pictures to better explain the diseases and conditions in question.

The advent of on-demand books makes us once again confront our traditional role—collecting books and journals. With per-article delivery of journals and on-demand books, bookstores and libraries and users are getting their materials "just in time." Traditionally, we have collected in a manner of "just in case." We ordered our books and journals with the studied knowledge of materials and our users needs. Then we put the materials on the shelves expecting our patrons to come by and use them. Perhaps "just in case" will not be adequate. The literature of librarianship offers many commentaries on our future (Bluh 1993). You can join the conversation. For example, the Medical Library Association has a collection development section. To read and/or contribute, you may join the online discussion group, Biomedical Library Acquisitions Bulletin (BLAB).

CATALOGING: INTRODUCTION

The books have been selected and ordered. They arrive in the library. Your next step is to supply the bibliographic control; it is time to catalog the books. Librarians have traditionally performed specialized roles in large libraries. The catalogers did the cataloging and nobody else did it. However, in a small library, you often have the opportunity to do a little bit of everything. One of the things that you will likely do is some cataloging. The intended purpose of cataloging is to make the materials in your collection retrievable in a systematic fashion. However, there is a bonus for the people who are doing the cataloging. If you spend part of your time with reference or collection development, your time spent cataloging will aid you in answering questions and knowing what is needed for the collection. If you are the only person in the library, you may not have a choice about whether you will be the one to do the cataloging. Some librarians feel that cataloging is to be avoided. Whether you enjoy it or not, cataloging is a great way to familiarize yourself with the subjects and works in your collection.

This chapter focuses on subject cataloging—the assigning of subject headings and classification numbers. Information retrieval is what health sciences libraries are about, and headings and classification numbers have been the main subject access points. Computerized catalogs can offer many more points for retrieval: words in the title, words from a corporate author, contents notes, and so on. This greatly enriches the catalog as an aid for our patrons. You will need to understand both subject cataloging and descriptive cataloging. Health sciences libraries do not differ from other libraries in cataloging techniques. A difference, however, will likely involve subject cataloging. To begin our look at cataloging in health sciences libraries, a look at the alternatives for classification and subject headings is in order.

NATIONAL LIBRARY OF MEDICINE CLASSIFICATION

There are two major classification schemes generally being used in libraries in the United States: Library of Congress (LC) and Dewey decimal. What classification system do medical libraries use? Many hospital libraries and medical school libraries use the National Library of Medicine scheme. This system is tailored specifically for biomedical publications. Other medical classifications, such as Cunningham classification and Boston Medical Library classification, have been used over the years. Many medical libraries that have used these other systems have switched to NLM, which offers several advantages.

1. Of the various classification systems dedicated to medicine, only NLM continues to be updated. The rest have not been revised in many years. Medicine is a dynamic field. Classifications need to grow, too. With the Boston system updated last in 1955 and Cunningham in 1967 and no further updates planned for either, these are not adequate (Scheerer and Hines 1974). Although new editions of NLM have not been published frequently, the current edition (1994) is the fifth.

2. The NLM system fits well with Library of Congress. Most medical libraries will need to collect materials that are not strictly medical. The library can use the LC system to classify nonmedical materials. Books on psychology, for example, may be conveniently classed in the *BF*'s. The Library of Congress has reserved for NLM the use of the *W*'s and *QT–QZ*. Meanwhile, the Library of Congress has its own classification for medicine, the *R*'s. Nonmedical libraries use the *R* schedule for their medical titles. Why would this not be sufficient for the medical libraries? The advantage can be seen in the way a special library often adapts a classification system to suit itself. If a whole organization and collection is dedicated to a particular topic (e.g., the lung), that topic's call number would be overwhelmed. Most of the books would be at one call number. The special library arranges to have a more detailed classification set aside for its primary subject. That is what happens with NLM, too, and with the part of the alphabet reserved for medicine. It can divide up the *W*'s more finely than the Library of Congress may have in mind for the *R*'s. You, in turn, may find the NLM call numbers too crowded in some of your specialties and may need to make your own adaptations to the NLM system.

3. An important factor in the choice has to do with the availability of cataloging information. Most of the cataloging done in libraries is not original cataloging. Libraries use cataloging copy they retrieve from the bibliographic utilities or other sources. Conveniently, many of these sources, such as the Online Computer Library Center (OCLC) and the Research Libraries Information

Network (RLIN), have cataloging information with both LC and NLM data. The availability of NLM catalog copy certainly makes that choice more appealing. The use of other classification systems will mean that you will need to do a lot more original cataloging or, at least, spend more time adapting other libraries' cataloging.

COMPARISON OF NLM AND LC SCHEDULES

Below are the call numbers in the 1994 NLM classification schedule along with their subjects. To the right are the LC call numbers that correspond to the NLM classification. Often a one-to-one correspondence for all aspects of these broad categories is not available. Look at the LC number listed as a location for much of the material in that subject. Note that *RC*, Internal Medicine, is a particularly crowded classification.

Preclinical Sciences

NLM Number	Subject	LC Number
QS	Human Anatomy	QM
QT	Physiology	QP
QU	Biochemistry	QP501
QV	Pharmacology	RM300
QW	Microbiology and Immunology	QR
QX	Parasitology	RC119
QY	Clinical Pathology	RB
QZ	Pathology	RB
Medicine and Related Subjects		
W	Health Professions	R690
WA	Public Health	RA421
WB	Practice of Medicine	R728
WC	Communicable Diseases	RC110
WD100	Nutrition Disorders	RC620
WD200	Metabolic Diseases	RC627.5
WD300	Immunologic and Collagen Diseases. Hypersensitivity	RC581
WD400	Animal Poisons	RA1255
WD500	Plant Poisons	RA1250
WD600	Diseases and Injuries Caused by Physical Agents	RC91

WD700	Aviation and Space Medicine	RC1030
WE	Musculoskeletal System	RC925
WF	Respiratory System	RC705
WG	Cardiovascular System	RC666
WH	Hemic and Lymphatic System	RC633
WI	Digestive System	RC799
WJ	Urogenital System	RC870
WK	Endocrine System	RC648
WL	Nervous System	RC321
WM	Psychiatry	RC435
WN	Radiology. Diagnostic Imaging	RM
WO	Surgery	RD
WP	Gynecology	RG
WQ	Obstetrics	RG
WR	Dermatology	RL
WS	Pediatrics	RJ
WT	Geriatrics. Chronic Disease	RC952
WU	Dentistry. Oral Surgery	RK
WV	Otorhinolaryngology	RF
WW	Ophthalmology	RE
WX	Hospitals and Other Health Facilities	RA960
WY	Nursing	RT
WZ	History of Medicine	R131

SUBJECT HEADINGS FOR BOOKS: MESH

There is also a choice to be made for the selection of subject headings. The medical librarian has a familiarity with MeSH (Medical Subject Headings) because IM and MEDLINE use MeSH for the indexing of articles. In the same way that the NLM classification is designed for medical libraries more adequately than the LC classification, MeSH has the advantage over the *Library of Congress Subject Headings* (Muench 1979). In addition, MeSH is updated every year. It would certainly make sense to use MeSH with the NLM classification. Before assuming that every medical collection should use NLM and MeSH, remember that large medical collections are often part of larger, general libraries. Thus cataloging for medical materials is integrated with the classification and subject headings used for the whole library (e.g., LC).

COPY CATALOGING

Most of the books you obtain have already been cataloged by some other library. This is of considerable help to you. You do not have to do original cataloging for most of the items you have. First, look for the existing cataloging record. Cataloging information may be found on the verso of the title page. This cataloging in publication (CIP) data is provided by the Library of Congress. Medical books usually include the NLM classification number and MeSH terms along with the LC classification number and subject headings. Other sources of medical cataloging information include CATLINE (now available on the Internet as Locator) and the NLM *Current Catalog*—sources discussed earlier in the chapter.

The bibliographic utilities OCLC and RLIN are important sources of cataloging information. These databases usually display the LC call number and subjects as well as the NLM call number and MeSH. The example displayed below is from a book titled *Diet, Nutrition, and Cancer: Directions for Research.*

Library of Congress	**National Library of Medicine**
RC262	QZ202
Cancer—nutritional aspects	Diet—adverse effects
Carcinogenesis	Neoplasms—etiology
	Nutrition

When you look at the Medical Subject Headings assigned to this book, you notice that they look similar to the terms used for journal articles. Additional rules apply to the cataloging of books. Also, the philosophy for book cataloging differs from the philosophy for journal cataloging. The subject headings applied to a full book typically number from one to four. Journal articles are much shorter than books but have two or three times as many subject headings. In medicine, the age of the patients is often important. To show the age aspect, additional subheadings are available to the cataloger that are not available to the indexer of articles: in infancy and childhood; in adolescence; in adulthood; in middle age; in old age. These headings look familiar. The indexing for MEDLINE has check tags for age groups (e.g., infant, child). For journal articles, separate MeSH headings are applied. For the cataloging of books, subheadings are used. Other subheadings are available to catalogers beyond the topical ones we have used. They are geographic, form, and language. One form of subheading, for example, is "popular works." Consult the *Annotated Alphabetic MeSH*, which includes "Cataloging Practices," a section that covers the use of headings and subheadings (National Library of Medicine 1994a).

ORIGINAL CATALOGING AND YOUR CATALOGING PHILOSOPHY

Many small medical libraries understand that their main responsibility, not surprisingly, is to serve their patrons. A small library has the flexibility to tailor cataloging to the needs of patrons. What, then, should be thought of the cataloging the librarian produces versus the cataloging in the bibliographic utilities? The bulk of the librarian's records will likely come from a cataloging utility. With the wide use of computers, it could very well be useful to have the records included in the bibliographic utility as well. A special library may have items not widely held at other libraries. To add them to the records, the librarian will need to verify that they meet the criteria for inclusion.

Our primary consideration is subject cataloging. However, we also need to give a thought to descriptive cataloging and the MARC record. The cataloging librarians in larger libraries do their cataloging with MARC. With the possibility of sharing records, the librarian in a small library will find it useful to understand the MARC record and consider using it for the online catalog.

AN EXERCISE IN ORIGINAL CATALOGING: SUBJECT CATALOGING

Some items that you want to have in your collection may not have copy catalog information. Reports that are authored by your own organization about your organization have usually not been cataloged elsewhere and are items you will want in your collection. For books without copy catalog information, what is your strategy? You will use what you have learned elsewhere about the form of the information that goes into the cataloging record. Your task is to assign subject headings and call numbers.

First, check to see if you have other books on this topic. Probably you do. What are their subject headings and call numbers? If you do not have any really similar items, what is the next step? You have the book in hand. It is *Arthropods and Human Skin*. Skimming through the book, you see that it is about disorders of the skin caused by insects and other arthropods. You go to your *Medical Subject Headings—Annotated Alphabetic List*. You see the heading "Insects" at B1.131.617+ and also "Arthropods" at B1.131+. In this case, the title word happens to fit well. The animals in question include a broader category than insects. We have always worried about specificity in our indexing of journal articles. That same principle applies in assigning subject headings to books. However, here the broader term is the appropriate one, so use "Arthropods" as one MeSH heading for this book. The book concerns itself with identifying the diseases of the skin, therefore assign this MeSH heading-subheading combination "Skin Diseases/Diagnosis." The problems are coming about due to bites and stings, and there happens to be a heading for that, "Bites and Stings." You now have three subject headings for your catalog. Now the question arises,

Where to shelve the book? Consult the *National Library of Medicine Classification*. This has a subtitle, *A Scheme for the Shelf Arrangement of Library Materials in the Field of Medicine and Its Related Sciences*. Take a look at the index. It uses *Medical Subject Headings* as entry points. "Bites and Stings" directs us to go to WD430; the WD400 section is for books on Animal Poisoning. "Skin Diseases" in the index directs us to the *WR* classification; *WR* is Dermatology. "Arthropods" presents us with some choices. First, the general section for "Arthropods" is QX460–570, Arthropods within the Parasitology category. Second, "Arthropods" has "Bites, Stings, and Poisoning," which takes us back to WD430. Third, "Arthropods" with "Cause of Skin Diseases" takes us to WR360–375. This part of the Dermatology category, *WR*, covers "Skin Diseases Caused by Arthropods." WR360 would seem to be a fitting place to shelve the book. Classification of books is often not completely satisfactory. A book may be about more than one subject, but it can be physically in only one place. You may identify the various subjects of the book with several subject headings. Try to classify the book to fit the subject of the book accurately and in a location you believe your patrons will look for it. This could easily mean that two libraries will shelve the same book at different call numbers. One more cautionary note on cataloging—this was just a brief look at subject cataloging. The descriptive cataloging and authority control of entries that you learn for general cataloging is needed in the health sciences libraries, too.

MISCELLANEOUS NOTES ON CATALOGING

Remember, you have a choice about the arrangement of your journals. Many large libraries catalog their serials. Most medical libraries arrange their journals in alphabetical order of the titles. There are very good reasons to catalog journals and assign call numbers (e.g., the not infrequent title changes). Your patrons will appreciate it if you at least shelve the current journals in alphabetical order by title.

As you catalog the new books, you add them to your catalog. Here is a question for both card catalogs and computerized catalogs. What do you do about superseded MeSH headings from the older books? Fredericksen and Michael (1976) wrote that many libraries did go through old cards and update—no small matter. There are many changes in headings each year. Along with many other reasons that a computerized catalog would be of interest, we can add this: It provides the capacity to make global changes or additions to our catalog records. Retrospective conversion of small collections is also not a daunting task. Organizations like MARCIVE, which have specialized in supplying the catalog cards for your traditional catalog, can also supply the machine readable data of your cataloging records.

As with indexing practices, cataloging practices need to be evaluated as we move to the online catalog. "The nature of subject searching is inexact and exploratory, a process of trying to match a user's information need, an author's intent and expertise, a subject heading list, and a subject cataloger's interpretation of all of these'' (Gregor and Mandel 1991: 46). Consistency in the cataloging process is a worthy goal. When users find the words that match the subject they have in mind, they have the key to much of the information. In the computerized environment, that goal may not be enough. In the old card catalog, users might find books with titles beginning with the words they have in mind. In addition, guide cards and ''see references'' are filed among the entries. For the online catalog, we need to do at least as much and perhaps more. Here are two suggestions. Guide users from their wording to the list of headings that might be relevant. Alternatively, the words users entered can be automatically mapped to the system's words, which then pull up the ''correct'' records without bothering (or informing?) the users. The lessons that have been learned from online searching of the abstracting and indexing services may be applicable to the catalog, too. We can take this opportunity to enrich our entries with abstracts or notes or even full text. You want to make this tool both useful and something people will use. Keep in mind that many patrons will avoid the catalog and confine their subject searching to the browsing of the shelves. This may not be the best search strategy because the book of interest could easily be in a different location on the shelf or the book may have been checked out.

When you set up your acquisitions and cataloging services, you may do things much differently than this chapter suggests. Your vendor of books may supply you with machine-readable cataloging records. Another recent trend involves ''outsourcing.'' For this, you contract the cataloging of your books to an outside company. A library cutting back on its expenses may find outsourcing more economical than hiring its own catalogers, with the expense of their salaries and benefits. Whether you do the cataloging yourself or your colleagues or staff do it or your book vendor supplies it or you employ an agency to do it, you need to understand the cataloging process. Cataloging is the way your collection of information is organized and, therefore, affects how it is retrieved.

5

Reference: Service and Sources

INTRODUCTION

The preface addressed the mission of the health sciences librarian, namely, to assist in the provision of good health care. An article title asks: "The Service Imperative: Do Library Services Improve the Quality of Patient Care?" (King 1989). We respond: "Yes, sure we do. Our work helps in the education of the health professionals. We find and transmit information that they need to use to make better decisions." How do we know this? How do we know that our activities actually have any impact on the patient? King maintains that we cannot effectively fulfill that role by merely accumulating all the journal citations that are on a topic and unloading the list on the health care provider. The individual responsible for direct patient care, the physician, needs usable information. He or she cannot utilize much of the literature on the particular subject being searched in the database. There are several reasons for this. Some of the literature is based on animal studies. The findings may eventually be helpful to the physician but are not currently ready to be used for the treatment of patients. Many published experiments do not use rigorous methodologies. For example, the selection of patients for different groups of a protocol may be random, or they may, instead, have unwittingly been influenced by the investigator. In the latter case, the physician will have less confidence in the results and not readily use that information. Therefore, although there is certainly a lot of literature out there that you can pass on to your patrons, much of it is not helpful to the practitioner. King says it is our role, our responsibility as librarians, to provide the "good," useful information and only the "good," useful information. This is not something we have always done, supplying this value added service.

The time has come for librarians to be more actively involved in meeting the needs of health care providers. Remember, too, your role as a special librarian. You do not always need to wait for your clientele to ask you for something. Your knowledge of the literature empowers you to provide information before patrons ask for it. Your task is to make their search easy for them. Whether you take on the responsibility of evaluating the literature, as noted above, or you do not, you can still make your patrons aware of information before they know they need it—before they even know it exists.

Providing reference service requires knowledge of the sources, and we will be looking at reference tools shortly. Another aspect of the reference process is to know your patrons. Most introductory reference courses in library school place great emphasis on the reference interview. Knowing that requestors often fail to ask clearly for the information they want, you must ask questions until you have ascertained specifically what they really want. To disregard this advice would not be correct. Indeed, you will find much written about it in any book on reference librarianship. But let's look more specifically at the interaction between you and your patrons. This interaction changes when you know them and their field of practice, as well as what their information-gathering practices have been in the past. You will often know not only what your patrons need but also what form they want the information to be in.

Let's look, for example, at Dr. Carpenter and Dr. Redman. Dr. Carpenter requests a computer search on lung cancer and smoking. That covers a tremendous amount of literature. It may seem that you really need, at least, a third parameter (e.g., females or passive smoking or something else to make the retrieval more manageable). However, you know Dr. Carpenter from your previous dealings with him. He wants just a few articles that are right on target within this general subject. He does not want to see citations mentioning these two ideas peripherally. A few recent articles, preferably review articles, are what he wants at this time. And he would like the abstracts, too. Next Dr. Redman drops in. He requests the last three years' worth of citations to studies using Fischer 344 rats. You have dealt with Dr. Redman many times. He does not care whether there are 700 citations on this or only seven. He wants to scan the titles—all of them. Removal of the foreign-language articles is in order, but he would like you to get a printout of the rest. If the number is large, print the titles only for him to scan. He may get back to you for the fuller citations for a dozen or two.

At this point, perhaps you want to advise the librarian: "You should have narrowed the topic to a few dozen titles in the first place by asking Dr. Redman what he really wanted. This is the reason for the reference interview, isn't it?" Yes, the reference interview would certainly be in order here for most requests. Retrieval can be limited in meaningful ways, and ordinarily you would use this technique. However, the point is this: Each person has different information needs and learning methods. Over time, it is true, costs for the information change, and then 700 citations or even titles might be prohibitively expensive. Now, though, you know Dr. Redman and what he wants, and you know Dr. Carpenter, too. There is nothing wrong in making suggestions that you believe will be helpful to serve the patron (e.g., narrow the topic, try a citation index). However, you do not need to impose an artificial structure on them just because you would do the search differently with another requestor who walks in the door. Standardization of service is not called for. Know your patrons and the sources.

THE NEED FOR INFORMATION

Clinicians need information. ''Investigators of the clinical problem-solving process have repeatedly shown the strong problem-specific performance of clinical problem solvers. Knowledge, not problem-solving strategy, is what differentiates expert from nonexpert performance'' (Connelly et al. 1990, 353). Physicians are good at solving problems (e.g., making diagnoses). What they need is more information. In a roundabout way, this supports the theme of today's medical schools. The emphasis is changing from memorizing the mountains of data in school to the development of problem-based learning and reasoning skills. Practicing physicians need to take in new data throughout their lives. Medical schools need to prepare students both by developing their problem-solving skills and by showing them how to be lifelong learners. It would be safe to say that both the information and the reasoning skills are needed. Researchers are in the same situation. In fact, they may need even more information. We can be a great help to them, as well. Here are a few clever words of advice to those researchers (it would be good if administrators responsible for library funding would hear them, too): ''Westheimer's Discovery: A couple of months in the laboratory can frequently save a couple of hours in the library'' (Crampon 1988, 41). Whether we are involved with helping clinicians make better decisions for their patients or saving researchers from reinventing the wheel (or unknowingly duplicating an experiment), the charge to us is clear: Get these people the information they need.

THE ATTITUDE OF THE REFERENCE LIBRARIAN

Although you can draw upon your experience to aid long-time patrons and have an established rapport with them, what is your attitude toward new requestors? Also, who are your patrons? So far in this book the patron has been classified as a health care provider or a researcher. Those categories may be your whole clientele. In other libraries, your role as a health sciences librarian will likely enable you to serve a broader group, the public. The theory of the reference interview seems to instruct you to take nothing for granted. It is almost as if to say, Do not give the patron the benefit of the doubt. This seems a bit arrogant regardless of who the patron is. Let's say the patron comes over to you hesitatingly (after working in a library for a while, a librarian often forgets that many people do not see libraries or librarians as friendly) and asks: "Where may I find the *Medical Journal of New England*?" More than one reference librarian would quickly reply: "You want the *New England Journal of Medicine*." It is a very sad commentary that librarians, medical or not, often seem to feel that nonlibrarians should know what we know. These librarians are sending the message "If we know, why don't you?" We then turn around and bemoan among ourselves that other people do not understand the worth of librarians. We cannot have it both ways. Either our knowledge base is trivial and we have little to offer, or we do have useful skills and knowledge and can be a great help to others. In this example, it may seem that the title in question must be the *New England Journal of Medicine*. Why should it be obvious to everybody who comes through the door? While you are at it, it might be worthwhile checking on the title that the patron gave to you. There could also be a *Medical Journal of New England*. Putting it bluntly, for a librarian there is something worse than being incompetent; it is being incompetent and arrogant. There is no excuse for belittling patrons or their requests, either in their presence or behind their backs.

FOLLOWING THE REFERENCE TRAIL

Here is one more diversion on our way to the sources. Dr. Delvecchio calls from the hospital. "Hello. We don't have much information at all on this. Could you help us? The title of the article is 'On the Origins of the Influencing Machine in Schizophrenia.' We think that the author's name is Trask and that is spelled *T r a s k*. The journal? Well, we really don't know. It could be *Psychoanalytic Annals*. That is just a guess. We think it was from the 1930s." This question can be answered quickly, you think. *Psychological Abstracts* (PA) has a cumulated author index for 1927–1958. Not many indexes have cumulations that cover so many years, and rarely will you see an electronic counterpart for data before the 1960s. A check of PA, however, finds no author by the name of Trask.

What to do next? The requestor was unsure of the date of the article. Often when the date of publication is unknown, it is convenient to use the citation index of the SCI. To appear in that index, an article does not have to have been written the year that you consult. It just has to have been cited that year. This is somewhat hit and miss, but with a lack of an abundance of cumulated indexes, it is a very useful and powerful source. By the way, *Cumulated Index Medicus* cumulates the months of one year and that is all. A check of a recent year of SCI shows that there is a Trask and there is the word "Origins" in the truncated title and it is a 1932 book. Parenthetically, although SCI only covers journals as citing references, the cited reference could be many things, including books.

This is exciting. A look in the library's catalog shows that we even own the book. The full title does not sound encouraging, but with all these positive elements in play—Trask, origins, the 1930s—a sense of satisfaction is felt as we head to the stacks. The title of the book is *Origin and Environment of Source Sediments of Petroleum.* This just does not seem a whole lot like the subject in question. The author is Parker Davies Trask. There is no sign of ''schizophrenia'' anywhere in this book on petroleum. Hmmmm. Let's check the contents again. No, there does not seem any way to bring ''schizophrenia'' into this book.

It is time to bite the bullet. This time, a look back at the subject index of the cumulated PA is the next step. There is an entry under ''Schizophrenia'' that has ''Influencing Machine'' in it. Moving along to the abstract, the citation is for a 1958 book, *Psychoanalysis*. It was published in France and is a collection of papers. This abstract very conveniently gives the contents. The last paper noted is ''V. Tausk, on the origin of 'the influencing machine' in schizophrenia.'' Now we have the author's name. A quick check of that cumulated author index yields the citation we want: ''Tausk, V. On the origin of the 'influencing machine' in schizophrenia. Psychoanal. Quar., 1933, 2, 519–556.'' The author's name was Tausk, not Trask, and the journal in question was *Psychoanalytic Quarterly* not *Psychoanalytic Annals.*

Was this the right way to handle this question? Perhaps not. This whole process took just ten minutes, but it was certainly not the direct route. Could not the subject index of the cumulated PA have been used in the first place? The information was there. Yes, it could have been. Perhaps there is another lesson here about our faith in subject indexing and why our patrons often go to a citation index instead of a subject index. This reference journey was not a textbook solution to the problem. However, was this fun? You bet it was. Was it satisfying getting the answer that the patron needed. Yes. Tracking down and finding the answers with dubious information was gratifying. The moral of this anecdote is that resourcefulness and persistence help a lot.

Before we leave the proselytizing section of this chapter, take a look at another example. An interlibrary loan request comes in for a book. You have the complete information: author, title, place of publication, publisher, year of publication, and the source of the citation. The date of publication is from seven years ago. You would like to verify the information given you by the patron and also identify the libraries that do own the book. You check RLIN, the Research Libraries Information Network. It is not there. You check OCLC, but it's not there. You check the *Cumulative Book Index*, *Books in Print*, and even *Index Medicus* and *Biological Abstracts.* You see no evidence of this publication as a book or even as a journal article. You call the publisher. They never published a book by that author with that title. That seems definitive. Remember, it is time consuming and difficult to prove a negative. This situation may come up every now and then for a book. However, researchers not infrequently want searches of the literature to yield negative results. Confident that nothing has been written on the topic in question, they want to be sure that nothing has been written on it. Your contribution is to join them in trying to prove that.

SAMPLING THE HEALTH SCIENCES REFERENCE TOOLS

The way to learn to use reference tools is to take questions and find answers. Tools should be thought of in categories in the same way you do for other reference tools. Is the person looking for an article in a journal? Does he or she need an address of an organization? Is a specific statistic called for? Experience will give you guidance in your choice of sources. Sometimes questions may be answered quickly by the first source you check. Often, more than one source needs to be consulted. Familiarize yourself with the print and electronic sources in order to efficiently handle many questions. This is a capability you will continuously want to expand. This section delineates specific categories of reference tools for the purpose of demonstrating the type of questions they will help answer. In most categories just two reference sources are illustrated here. Look at these as representatives only. They may not be the most useful tools to you. For fuller description of many tools you should be familiar with, consult *Introduction to Reference Sources in the Health Sciences* (Roper and Boorkman 1994). Remember, also, the books on the more general reference materials. The following sections include citations to the literature to guide you to more information about the tools. However, the reference item itself (e.g., *Index to Scientific and Technical Proceedings*) does not appear in the bibliography of this book. In most cases, you will want to go to the reference tool to read the introductory material that explains its scope and layout and to examine its entries and indexes.

DIRECTORIES—BIOGRAPHIES

Regardless of the type of library you work in, you will get many questions about the qualifications of individual physicians. This question could come from a health care professional but is often from a family member or patient checking on the credentials of a physician under consideration. A related request is one not just for information concerning education and experience but for a recommendation of a physician. True, some publications claim to list "best doctors." Consider, however, referring that question to the local medical society. We should provide insight about the timeliness or authority of our published sources, but our role does not include recommendations of health care providers. For the straightforward questions on the education or experience of a physician, our directories supply some basic information. The AMA *Directory of Physicians in the United States* published its thirty-fourth edition in 1994 with information on 686,000 physicians. Before the thirty-third edition, the directory was entitled

American Medical Directory, with the subtitle *Directory of Physicians in the United States, Puerto Rico, Virgin Islands, and U.S. Physicians Temporarily Located in Foreign Countries*. The directory maintains that coverage today, and although this directory is a publication of the AMA, a physician does not have to be a member of AMA to be included. In this four-volume directory, most physicians are given just one line of coded information. An alphabetical index of names of physicians directs you to the state and city of that physician. Under the city is the full information displayed in coded form. For example, in volume 4 at Rhode Island and Providence, one of the listings is this:

STEPHENS, Karl Frederick, 110 LOCKWOOD ST 02903 #024–07 L67 OPH *020 +35

The name and the address are clear. The code for the medical school Dr. Stephens attended is "#024–07"—Tufts University School of Medicine, Boston. "L67" is for the year he was licensed to practice medicine in Rhode Island. "OPH" for ophthalmology is the physician's designation of his primary field of practice. "*020" means that direct patient care is his type of practice. This directory includes physicians whether they are certified medical specialists or not. "+35" signifies that Dr. Stephens is certified by the American Board of Ophthalmology.

The Official ABMS Directory of Board Certified Medical Specialists is a product of both the American Board of Medical Specialties (ABMS) and Marquis Who's Who. For several years, both organizations published their own listings. Their consolidation began with the twenty-sixth edition. Before that, the separate titles were the *ABMS Compendium of Certified Medical Specialists* and the *Directory of Medical Specialists*. To be included, the physician must have become certified by one of the 24 medical specialty boards. Therefore, this directory includes a subset of the physicians found in the *Directory of Physicians in the United States*. Compare this entry for Dr. Stephens with the preceding one:

STEPHENS, Karl F.
Cert Oph 70. b 38 Providence RI. MD Tufts U 62. Int Rot 62–63 (Hosp U Penn Philadelphia) Res Oph 65–68 (Mass EE Infirm Boston).
Cur Hosp Appt (RI Hosp, Providence RI). Clin Asst Prof Oph Surg (Brown U). AAOph–AMA–AOA–NEOS. FT-Priv Prac Solo. 110 Lockwood St 02903–4801 (401) 421–3867.

More information is included, and the entries are less cryptic. You could read most of this entry without having to look at the list of abbreviations at the front of the volume for translations. Spelled out, the entry would read like this:

STEPHENS, Karl F. Certified in Ophthalmology in 1970. Born in 1938, Providence, RI. Medical Degree from Tufts University, 1962. Internship, 1962–63 at the Hospital, University of Pennsylvania, Philadelphia. Residency in Ophthalmology, 1965–68, at the Massachusetts Eye and Ear Infirmary, Boston. Current Hospital Appointment, Rhode Island Hospital, Providence, RI. Academic Appointment, Clinical Assistant Professor, Ophthalmologic Surgery, Brown University. Professional Memberships: American Academy of Ophthalmology, American Medical Association, Alpha Omega Alpha, and New England Ophthalmological Society. Full-Time Private Practice Solo. [Also office address and telephone number.]

DIRECTORIES—ORGANIZATIONS

Along with requests for information about people are many questions about organizations relating to biomedicine. Hospitals, not surprisingly, are among the organizations of interest. In a survey of medical school reference librarians by Johnson and others (1990), the publication mentioned most often as essential was the *American Hospital Association Guide to the Health Care Field* [Chicago, American Hospital Association, annual]. This is a directory that gives a lot of information in compact and coded arrangements. A hospital address can be found here. The size of a hospital, measured by number of beds, is also here. Fairly detailed information for services offered is included. For instance, from the 1994 directory you can determine which hospitals in Milwaukee, Wisconsin, have the extracorporeal shock-wave lithotripter (facility code number 16). St. Luke's Medical Center is one. Information on which agencies accredit the hospital, the level of occupancy, and other administrative data are also given.

The *Medical and Health Information Directory* [Detroit, Gale Research, 7th ed., 1994] comes in three volumes: 1. Organizations, Agencies, and Institutions; 2. Publications, Libraries, and Other Information Resources; and 3. Health Services. A variety of organizations are included in this set. Much of the information may be found in Gale's other publications (e.g., *Encyclopedia of Associations*). However, the variety, extensiveness, and convenience of this set make it very useful. For instance, would you like to know (1) the state association in Vermont for lupus erythematosus; (2) the address of the dental board in Arkansas; (3) the schools of optometry; (4) the audiovisual producers in the health care field; (5) the eye banks in Wisconsin; (6) a listing of multiple sclerosis clinics? The variety of references to associations, organizations, services, and publications provides answers to many questions.

DIRECTORIES—MEETINGS

Informal and formal exchanges of information are vital to the scientific endeavor. One conduit of the formal and informal flow of information is the scientific meeting. Numerous organizations bring their memberships together regularly, including library organizations (e.g., Medical Library Association, American Library Association). There are thousands of science associations, and different types of publications may come from their meetings. Preprints of papers to be presented may be available, or the conference program may contain abstracts of the papers. In addition, the full papers of some or all of the presentations given at a meeting may be published in book form after the meeting. (Note that the book may be published a long time after the meeting is held.) Abstracts or full papers may appear in an issue of the journal of the society that sponsored the meeting. We need to find information about meetings both before and after they take place. People who make plans to attend meetings need to know the particulars. Patrons want to track down the information that had been presented at meetings.

World Meetings—United States and Canada and *World Meetings—Outside United States and Canada* [New York, Macmillan Publishing Company, bimonthly] are publications giving information on upcoming meetings. Their coverage is not limited to biomedicine and science. Meetings may be found by subject (keyword), date, location, publication (where the proceedings will be published), deadline date for submission of abstract for the program, and name of sponsoring organization. Therefore, for instance, if you wanted to attend a meeting next year in Cincinnati, Ohio, here is a place in which you might find one.

Quite often you will have requests for papers that were presented at a meeting. The patron wants to know if the proceedings—the papers from that meeting—were ever published. In Chapter 4 we examined reasons (cost, quality, etc.) why many do not buy these published conference proceedings. However, people do use them, so we need to buy or borrow them. First we need to discover if the proceedings we require have been published. The information the patron provides may include any of the following: the author's name, the title of the paper, the title of the meeting, the sponsoring organization of the meeting, the editor of the proceedings, and the place and date of the meeting. A very useful tool for locating the proceedings with any of several entry points is *Index to Scientific and Technical Proceedings* [Philadelphia, Institute for Scientific Information, monthly]. This tool includes the following indexes: (1) category index (broad subject of the meeting); (2) author and editor index (includes all the authors of all the papers published in the proceedings); (3) sponsor index (the scientific or other association or organization); (4) meeting location index; (5) permuterm subject index (an index to all the words in every meeting title and every title of all the papers published within those meetings; same type of index as found in the SCI. See Chapter 2); and (6) corporate author indexes arranged by state and name of organization. This tool is especially useful because of the numerous entry points.

This is the question your patron has: ''I have this information about a paper presented at a meeting in Cleveland a few years ago. Unfortunately, the only things I know are the author of the paper and title of the paper: G. J. Alfano and 'The Role of the Family in the Rehabilitation of the Elderly.' '' You cannot go to the library catalog to find this; it is a paper from a meeting, and you do not know which meeting. There is a chance that you may find this in an index to the journal literature if the papers of a meeting were published as part of a journal. Were that the case, you could easily find this from the author's name. If that is not the case, a check of the *Index to Scientific and Technical Proceedings* is in order. You can look through a few years in the author or title word indexes. A check of the 1990 index leads us directly to the article in question. It was from the tenth Annual Fall Symposium on Practicing Rehabilitation with Geriatric Patients, Cleveland, Ohio, October 13–14, 1988. In 1990 Springer Publishing Company published the proceedings in a book.

DIRECTORIES—EDUCATION

You will have many questions about medical education as well as for other programs in the health sciences. After a student earns a medical degree from a medical school, he or she needs to find a program in which to do residency. For many years the publication used for this purpose was the *Directory of Residency Training Programs.* The name changed to the *Graduate Medical Education Directory* [Chicago, American Medical Association, annual], but the color of the cover, green, remained the same. A more important change also occurred. This information may now be obtained through the AMA's interactive program, AMA FREIDA. FREIDA stands for Fellowship and Residency Electronic Interactive Database Access. The FREIDA menu system guides searchers to construct their own sets of ''hits.'' Searchers specify (1) what specialty they are intent on pursuing, (2) what part of the country they would like to reside in, (3) what size hospital they want to work in, (4) what facilities they would like the hospital to have, and so on. The capability of manipulating the data is a big advantage FREIDA has over the AMA's ''Green Book.'' The 1995 FREIDA has information from the programs current as of August 1, 1994. The student would ordinarily use FREIDA himself or herself and be lead through it with a search like this: ''FREIDA welcomes you and asks you to select a medical specialty.'' Codes are displayed, and you choose ''141, Internal Medicine—Cardiovascular Disease.'' Next, you select which region or state you wish to go to. You select ''ENC, East North Central'' (the Midwest). There are 29 programs that meet these criteria. The list may be narrowed further with several more options. For instance, you may select the size of the program (e.g., ''1–10 positions'' has seven programs; ''11–20 positions,'' fifteen programs). Additional parameters allow you to narrow the list further if you wish.

The *Allied Health Education Directory* [Chicago, American Medical Association, annual] is a source that briefly describes a number of health care occupations and provides information on accredited educational programs. The 26 jobs include, among others, cytotechnologists, emergency medical technicians and/or paramedics, medical laboratory technicians, and physical therapists. Did you need to know if there are any programs in medical record administration in Nebraska? The College of Saint Mary has one in Omaha. What are the prerequisites for and curriculum of an accredited radiation therapy technologist program? That information is here also.

HANDBOOKS

The venerable *CRC Handbook of Chemistry and Physics* [Boca Raton, FL, CRC Press, annual] will be consulted a lot by your patrons for information ranging from melting points of an inorganic compound to the molecular weight of an organic substance. Closer to the biomedical realm are the handbooks published by the Federation of American Societies for Experimental Biology. The *Biology Data Book* series contains information ranging from the life spans of various animals, to the number of chromosomes of selected organisms, to the average weight of the human spleen. Unlike the *CRC Handbook of Chemistry and Physics*, many handbooks are not frequently updated. Some facts may not be expected to change, but others will. Keep that in mind in your use of the handbooks in biology with an eye out for computer accessible ''handbooks.''

DRUG INFORMATION

Questions to be answered by handbooks may not be that frequent in your library. Requests for information on drugs, in contrast, will be continuous. There are many sources for this information, too. The *Physicians Desk Reference* (PDR) [Oradell, NJ, Medical Economics Co., annual] is widely held by libraries, physicians, and others. Librarians are usually told that this source may not be as complete or unbiased as some other drug sources. The descriptions of drugs in the PDR are the same as those the drug companies include in the packaging of the drugs. Therefore, these descriptions contain information that the Food and Drug Administration (FDA) rules must be there. It may be argued that since these descriptions come from the drug manufacturers themselves, other sources should be kept in mind, too. The PDR does have to include such things as indications, effects, dosages, contraindications, and adverse reactions. It is also noteworthy that this and other drug books list adverse effects in abundance. Seemingly, every possible effect makes its way onto the list.

Whereas the PDR has its emphasis on descriptions of specific drugs, the *Drug Evaluations Annual* focuses on drug groups and includes discussions on ''the basic pharmacologic information, principles of therapeutics, pathogenesis or diagnosis of disease to the extent deemed necessary to facilitate the use of drugs in patients, and comparative drug evaluations within a pharmacologic or therapeutic category'' (American Medical Association 1995, iii). This is now published each year and has updates available during the year. The United States Pharmacopeial Convention publishes the *USP Dispensing Information* (USP DI) in two separate volumes: *Drug Information for the Health Care Professional* and *Advice for the Patient: Drug Information in Lay Language*. Updates are provided throughout the year for the USP DI, too.

Databases for drug information are available. Updated information is essential here, and computer updating and access fit in well with that need. The variety of applications range from the online databank, to the CD-ROM, to the PDR with an electronic display that fits in the palm of your hand—or the doctor's hand as he or she moves through the hospital. Related to drug information is the need for data on toxicology and poisoning. There are sources for these, also, but the best tool is the telephone. Poison Control Centers throughout the country are accessible by telephone.

DICTIONARIES AND ENCYCLOPEDIAS

Dorland's Illustrated Medical Dictionary, cited in Chapter 2, is one of the authorities for the usage of IM terms. Because medical dictionaries will get a lot of use in your library, you will want to have a few on hand. There are two types of arrangements of medical dictionaries. Some dictionaries, like *Dorland's*, take a classified or inverted approach. For example, if you were looking for ''aplastic anemia,'' you'd need to look under the heading ''anemia,'' not under ''aplastic.'' Other dictionaries have the more natural-language order entry ''aplastic anemia.'' Medical dictionaries come in several levels—for the physician, for the nurse or allied health worker, and for the lay public. Some dictionaries have American spelling, others British spelling.

Unlike the situation with dictionaries, up-to-date and useful encyclopedias in biology and medicine have been difficult to find. Perhaps the fast pace of the field and the time and effort to produce an encyclopedia make it too difficult to have a timely encyclopedic source. However, an encyclopedia in medicine and biology would have a large audience. Students and interested lay people would like to have meaningful, well-rounded, understandable presentations of today's biomedical topics. Academic Press has published some encyclopedias in the last few years: *Encyclopedia of Human Biology* (8 volumes), *Encyclopedia of Microbiology* (4 volumes), and *Encyclopedia of Immunology* (3 volumes).

GOVERNMENT DOCUMENTS AND TECHNICAL REPORTS

For federally funded projects, at least, the investigators must prepare and submit to the funding agency the reports of the progress they have made. These may take the form of quarterly reports, annual reports, or final reports. They may be skimpy, or they may be substantive. Many times the reports are extensive. The technical report may be the fullest public disclosure of the details and results of the experiment because the editor of the subsequent journal article will trim much of that data. Therefore, although the technical report is not nearly as widely read as the journal article, it may be a very useful document. Because technical reports are not available through the normal publication sources, they have been included in the designation "the gray literature." The report goes to the funding agency, and a copy of the report is sent to the National Technical Information Service (NTIS). Significantly, once the report reaches NTIS, it is always available. It never goes out of print. For a comparatively moderate price, you can order any report ever sent to NTIS.

Two types of publications that do not come from the traditional, commercial publishers may be crudely divided this way: (1) those originating from the federal government and (2) those that are distributed by the government but are produced by government contractors. Documents from the legislative, judicial, and executive branches are often handled by the superintendent of documents and the U.S. Government Printing Office. These publications are often part of the depository system and found in the *Monthly Catalog of United States Government Publications.*

To identify those thousands of technical reports from government contractors, you need the *Government Reports Announcements and Index.* A patron comes to the reference desk and points to a reference at the end of a journal article. It reads "W. L. Hanson. Testing of Experimental Compounds for Efficacy against Leishmania. AD-A229 734/9." This is not an article in a journal, although the information may later find its way into a journal. It is not a book. It is a report prepared, in this case, by the Georgia University Research Foundation. This report as well as all the reports for the last forty years that have been indexed in *Government Reports Announcements and Index* are available from NTIS in Springfield, Virginia. Often the key to locating the publication, and sometimes the only information that you are presented with, is the report number. The *Government Reports Announcements and Index* has a report number index as well as a personal author index, corporate author index, keyword index, and contract number index. In the 1980s a move was made to privatize NTIS, which is part of the Department of Commerce. It may be noted that most of the work reported in the millions of documents was funded by government money, and that the government operation of NTIS has guaranteed continuous access to all the publications. With NTIS, not only will you be able to identify the publication your patron wants but you will be able to get it. Over the coming years we expect electronic access to the full text of much of the journal literature that we use. It will be convenient. However, having the electronic full-text access of government documents and technical reports should mean unprecedented use of that gray literature.

INFORMATION ON JOURNALS

Many questions will come to you about journals. Do you own this journal? Why don't you have that journal? Which library near here has this journal? You have numbers 1, 2, 4, and 5 on the shelf? Where is number 3? You will receive questions with incomplete journal titles and questions with journal titles abbreviated in unconventional ways. Various sources can help you identify the journals. One very useful tool is the *Chemical Abstracts Service Source Index* (CASSI), which has information on publications indexed in *Chemical Abstracts*. Whereas IM covers over 3,000 journals and BIOSIS has over 6,000 serials, *Chemical Abstracts* includes over 15,000 publications. Fields beyond chemistry are covered (e.g., biology and medicine). Although *Chemical Abstracts* does not have all that is in IM and BA, its coverage is great. The entries are alphabetized by their CASSI abbreviation. Therefore, for instance, the *Australian Journal of Pharmaceutical Sciences* is alphabetized AUSTJPHARMSCI, with those letters of the titles in bold type. When you have an obscure abbreviation to identify, often CASSI is just the thing. It is convenient to have a source that shows you that Ann. Med. Exp. Biol. Fenn. is *Annales Medicinae Experientalis et Biologiae Fenniae*. Also noteworthy is that although coverage among the abstracting and indexing services overlaps, there is no guarantee that they will abbreviate the same title the same way. Unlike most lists of journals that accompany the abstracting and indexing services, CASSI also gives locations of libraries around the country that own each title.

SERLINE (SERials onLINE), a database on the MEDLARS system, includes information on about 80,000 biomedical serials. This covers journals well beyond what are indexed for MEDLINE and even beyond the holdings of NLM itself. SERLINE is now available on the Internet in Locator. Because you will get many questions concerning serials—for interlibrary loan, for purchase of a title, or for verification of a citation that goes in a paper, for example—sources on serials will be well used in your library.

TRANSLATIONS

Fortunately for many of us in North America, English is the language of medicine. It is notable that in many countries in which the native language is not English, biomedical scientists often publish their articles in English. Even the journals that are published in those countries, including official publications of professional societies, often include only English-language articles. Here are some examples: *Archives Internationales de Pharmacodynamie et de Therapie* (from Belgium), *Acta Psychiatrica Scandinavica* (from Sweden), and *Acta Pathologica Japonica* (from the Japanese Society of Pathology). For a closer look at this point, see "The Development of English as an International Language of Medicine" (Maher 1986).

To be sure, many biomedical articles are still written in languages other than English. When you look at an issue of IM, quite a number of titles are in brackets. Your patrons may want to obtain these articles, anyway. With the limited foreign-language capabilities of the North American biomedical scientist, this poses some potential problems. Languages not using the Roman alphabet (e.g., Russian and Japanese) present particular difficulties. Because it is expensive to get an on-demand translation, you need to determine if the article has already been translated into English. Some journals are conveniently available as cover-to-cover English translations from their native tongue. This has most frequently involved Russian journals. If you do not subscribe to one of the journals in translation (they are very expensive), the articles may be obtained through the regular interlibrary loan channels. To search for translations of articles not in the cover-to-cover translations, you can next go to an index of translations, *World Translations Index* [Delft, Netherlands, International Translations Centre, ten issues per year]. The publication is a result of the merging of indexes and title changes of *World Transindex* and *Translations Register-Index.* Use the subject access, author index, or an index that uses the journal title, year, volume, issue, and pages. There is one attribute that this tool has in common with the SCI citation index. A publication may never be cited or may be cited many years after its initial publication. An article written in 1975 may be translated at any time from 1975 to the present, or it may never be translated at all. For those articles found with translations, information is given on how to acquire them. The cost will likely be a bit higher than an interlibrary loan but much less than an on-demand translation.

CONSUMER HEALTH INFORMATION

Many traditional health sciences libraries have not acquired very much material in consumer health. They have left that to public libraries. As funding for institutions decreases, the directions of organizations may change as well. For instance, most acute care hospitals have concentrated on the traditional concerns of medicine, namely, treating people after they have become sick. They have not usually exercised much leadership in the consumer health movement and preventive medicine. This is changing as hospitals have been looking into additional ways to generate revenue, and some are reaching out to the consumers and to wellness programs. With their more extensive information resources, medical school libraries can provide valuable services here, too (La Rocco 1994). Some of our standard literature, prominent medical journals, have been recommended for public library collections (Spurlock and Kovacs 1986). For health sciences libraries, however, we need to expand into other types of materials to meet that need. The *Consumer Health Information Source Book* [Phoenix, Oryx, 1994] and *Managing Consumer Health Information Services* [Phoenix, Oryx, 1991], both by Alan Rees, are good sources for the library to start with. There is also *Health Index* on CD-ROM from Information Access Company, which focuses on lay-level coverage.

Even if we have not been collecting information intended for the public, we have been receiving questions from them. In fact, the public is likely to call us because of our expertise and our collection compared to the public library. How should we be handling those medical questions? Many health sciences librarians do not encounter the sensitive issues that the public librarian knows well. Working with health care professionals, there is no problem of censorship. The librarian feels no restraint in passing along to the professional, for example, information about a poor prognosis of a disease. What does the librarian do when the question about a fatal illness comes from the patient or the family of the patient? There are a few things you should keep in mind. You are not in the position of keeping information from people. It is your duty to deliver the information people are requesting. From the Medical Library Association (MLA) ''Code of Ethics for Health Sciences Librarians'': ''Society—The health sciences librarian promotes access to health information for all and creates and maintains conditions of freedom of inquiry, thought, and expression that facilitate informed health care decisions. . . . Profession—The health sciences librarian conducts all professional relationships with courtesy and respect'' (Medical Library Association 1995, 56). The request may involve a sensitive and tragic problem, and we are human beings, too. Is it our role when getting a telephone call to tell the caller that the books indicate that their illness is almost always fatal? The situation does not have to be handled in that way. There are appropriate ways to do this. The librarian should emphasize the need for the patient to talk to his or her physician because the specifics of the case need to be taken into account. Also, there are limitations of the published information. Whether you are passing along prognoses of diseases or side effects of drugs, you should clearly explain the fallibility of the information, the possibility of discoveries since publication, as well as potential irrelevance for the patient's circumstances. This is applicable with any reference work, but it is most important here, where one is dealing with matters of life and death.

GUIDES TO THE LITERATURE

The Rees source book just mentioned is a guide to the literature of the consumer health field. Barbara Smith Shearer and Geneva L. Bush, *Finding the Sources of Medical Information: A Thesaurus-Index to the Reference Collection* [Westport, CT, Greenwood, 1985], have compiled a useful book to direct you to the specific medical texts and reference books you will need to answer a question. Their text lists 447 publications by title. Next is an author index. After that is the actual entry point, the ''thesaurus-index.'' One entry in the index has the heading ''Vital Statistics, U.S.'' Under that are broader terms, narrower terms, and related terms that you may choose to check. Then numbers are given to the titles of publications that fit the category (e.g., 436—*Vital and Health Statistics Series*). Another guide to the literature has been compiled by Mary Glen Chitty, *Federal Information Sources in Health and Medicine* [New York, Greenwood, 1988]. Since this guide is about finding government publications and sources outside the traditional book and journal publications, this should be very helpful in finding materials and information.

STYLE MANUALS

The literature of your patrons is the journal. They will be writing articles that they wish to have published. Often they are looking for the guidelines for submission of articles for specific journals. There are general style guides available: the AMA *Manual of Style* [Baltimore, Williams & Wilkins, 8th ed., 1989] and the *Scientific Style and Format: the CBE Manual for Authors, Editors, and Publishers* [New York, Cambridge University Press, 6th ed., 1994]. There are also recommendations from the Vancouver Group, which originated from a meeting of several editors in Vancouver, British Columbia, in 1978. These guidelines were intended to standardize certain elements of the scientific paper. They were not intended to take the place of each journal's "Instructions for Authors," and they certainly have not. For one thing, there are so many seemingly pointless variations in the ways journals want the references to cite articles listed. Take just the author part: P. D. Jones; PD Jones, P D Jones; Jones, P. D.; Jones P D; Jones PD; P. D. JONES; and so on. Then there are the variations on journal abbreviations. Authors who are unsuccessful in the submission of the manuscript to one journal have the added inconvenience of changing the style to fit the next journal to which they submit their paper. Actually, some bibliographic software packages, such as Reference Manager, are designed to address just this problem. With a touch of a key or two or three, the citation format can be changed to the requirements of the next journal. A useful publication, too, is *National Library of Medicine Recommended Formats for Bibliographic Citation* [Bethesda, MD, National Library of Medicine, 1991].

HEALTH STATISTICS

The preceding sections present insufficient sketches of reference areas and their sources. A slightly more detailed discussion for one reference area is reserved here for health statistics. Many of the statistics requested will be concerning diseases. It is therefore worthwhile for you to understand some basic concepts that apply to these statistics (Palmore and Gardner 1983). "Incidence" is the rate of occurrence. How many people of population X contracted disease A in year Z. This is related to but not the same concept as "prevalence," or how widespread disease A is in year Z. The prevalence of the disease is the percentage of the population that has that disease in that time period. You will want to understand different measurements of mortality, fertility, and so on.

Supplying numerical information to requestors may be a time-consuming and difficult task. Frequently the numbers that people are seeking are not included in your handful of standardized statistical sources (e.g., *Statistical Abstract of the United States*. (The *Statistical Abstract* takes data from other sources, i.e., abstract.) There are several reasons for this. The requestor needs more specific information (e.g., how many people have a certain disease at specific ages in that part of the country). Another cause for the difficulty of finding the statistics is that the information is not collected very often. For many diseases and other concerns, there is no firm interval for collection. Statistics may not be collected annually or every fifth year or every tenth year. According to Dr. David Rogers:

> In health care, even fairly simple statistics are not regularly collected, or when they are, they are processed so slowly that they are not available until two to five years after the fact. Thus in most communities no one knows how often individuals are seen by their doctors or how many mothers are receiving pregnancy care or whether the changes we are making in . . . the delivery of care are resulting in more or fewer infant deaths or deaths from heart disease or cancer or diabetes or what-have-you. (Cohn 1989, 148)

Just a few diseases are notifiable. For those, physicians are directed to report the diseases to the local department of health. These are likely to be communicable diseases such as tuberculosis. Other ailments that people have keen interests in are not set up to be reported by physicians. The occurrences of the diseases you are looking for are tabulated by surveys and sampling and the use of statistical extrapolation. An example of this can be seen with ongoing publications of the National Center for Health Statistics, *Vital and Health Statistics*. The published data in these have the two attributes from above. The information comes from surveys and is typically gathered and published at uneven intervals. Take the National Health and Nutrition Examination Survey (NHANES). (NHANES is also referred to as N-HANES or HANES.) This survey is large and expensive (Marwick 1990). HANES I was conducted from 1971 to 1975, and HANES II was 1976–1980. HANES III began in 1988. *Vital and Health Statistics* has published information from the studies at irregular intervals. Consequently, it is often not a simple matter to provide the exact information needed and with the specific time period requested. Walsh and Bothmer (1991) have compiled a reference tool to help get at the information, *Vital and Health Statistics Series: An Annotated Checklist and Index to the Publications of the Rainbow Series* [Westport, CT: Greenwood, 1991]. Note that *Vital and Health Statistics* includes several series. For example, Series 13 is *Data from the National Health Survey*. Number 122 of Series 13 is *Detailed Diagnoses and Procedures, National Hospital Discharge Survey*, 1993 [Hyattsville, MD: National Center for Health Statistics, 1995].

Some publications do come out regularly. *Statistical Abstract* is an annual and may be found in almost all libraries. Others sources may be found in many libraries. Still others may be expensive and not sufficiently used in a small library to warrant the purchase or subscription. However, you will need to be familiar with all those sources whether you own them or not. The government publishes great varieties of statistical information that do not always find their way into handbooks. The *American Statistics Index* and also the *Statistical Reference Index* (for nonfederal government and nongovernmental sources) are indispensable tools. These certainly are not limited to biomedicine, but they are very useful for us. The Congressional Information Service publishes those as well as the *Index to Health Information.*

Another important source is your telephone. Some information is collected but not published or not widely disseminated. Organizations that monitor individual diseases are good sources for you to utilize. For instance, the American Cancer Society or the American Heart Association—the national organizations or the local organizations—should be remembered and utilized as well as governmental organizations. Remember, too, trade associations and other private sector sources. For example, a patron needed to know the average dimensions of the human armpit. The information was not in the *Biology Data Book* or other traditional sources. The librarian called a deodorant manufacturer and got the answer (Lavendel 1977).

COMPUTER ACCESS TO STATISTICS

Most of the databases we have used have been bibliographic. We can search our regular bibliographic databases for statistics and search *American Statistics Index* (paper, online, or CD-ROM). Health statistics directly available online will make them much easier to get to and more widely used. An example of a data database that we have had access to for several years is Registry of Toxic Effects of Chemical Substances. The database contains the values for toxicity, not just the pointer to the book that has the information. Social scientists have been regular users of such databases. Census data online provides not only a handy way to get at a lot of statistics but also allows the user to combine and juxtapose data in ways that had not been done by the data gatherers. We can connect into those types of sources, too. For a list of some of them, see "A Compendium of Public Health Data Sources" (Gable 1990). Agencies housing this data include the National Center for Health Statistics, National Institute of Occupational Safety and Health, Food and Drug Administration, Centers for Disease Control (CDC), Health Care Financing Administration, Bureau of the Census, Bureau of Labor Statistics, and the U.S. Department of Agriculture. The CDC system has developed WONDER (Friede, Reid, and Ory 1993).

THE RELIABILITY OF SOURCES

Core collections of standard medical books were discussed in Chapter 4. In each field of medicine, there are books that are regarded as authoritative. Students learn from them, and practicing physicians consult them. New editions are published every few years. Some of them (e.g., *Scientific American Medicine*), are arranged in looseleaf or CD-ROM formats to allow for more regular updating. Physicians are acutely aware of the rapid advance of knowledge. Textbooks, we understand, are out of date. Knowing that the findings and advice of one edition are sometimes rejected in the next, how do we respond toward the literature and to the authority of the literature? First of all, we do strive to acquire and disseminate current information. You can work only with what currently exists. However, it would seem wise to keep a skeptical mind. A drug may be found to be harmful. A routine operation may later be seen to yield long-term difficulties. ''But all any scientist can scientifically say—say with certainty in almost any such case—is, there is a very strong probability that such and such is true. . . . Widely believed theories or conclusions are often proved wholly or partly wrong. . . . Scientists are often wrong. In science this is not necessarily a failing'' (Cohn 1989, 9). Along with the limitations of current knowledge, there is the reality of human error as well as the possibility of fraud (more on that in Chapter 7).

FINDING THE PRE-PRIMARY LITERATURE: BEFORE THE JOURNAL ARTICLE

Laboratory notebooks have the initial written record and contain the most complete information on an experiment. The methods are spelled out, and the daily notes are there. The raw data, those measurements gathered with the laboratory equipment, are also supposed to be there. The observations, results, and summaries are noted. Unfortunately, the laboratory notebooks are not usually part of the public record. After all, the basis of science is its reproducibility. A researcher specifies his or her methods with the assumption that another scientist using the same type of experiment and resources can achieve the same results. This, in practice, cannot happen very often. It takes a great amount of time and money to do most studies. A scientist is not going to give up valuable time to merely confirm someone else's discovery. The glory goes to the first discoverer, anyway. Therefore findings from that original research will more or less stand on their own until confirmed or refuted by a related study that may be funded and completed later on. Were the laboratory notebooks available, others would see the experiment in its greatest detail. It should be remembered that errors may creep into an experiment even if the proposed methodology is sound. Human beings conduct the research. Errors will happen. Unless there is a great fuss over possible fraud, the information in laboratory notebooks may never be seen by outsiders. ''Scientific publications tell only part of the story, and if laboratory notebooks were examined more often, it is likely that people would learn more about the process of discovery'' (Altman 1995, C1). This is a gap in the stream of scientific information.

REFERENCE SERVICE AND THE JOURNAL LITERATURE

We have seen that much of the literature is not usable. More specifically, it is not useful for the physician treating a patient. Although many types of publications were covered in the last several pages, we always seem to get back to the journal literature. Chapter 3 included suggestions for searching MEDLINE for papers from clinical trials or randomized controlled trials or meta-analysis studies. Haynes (1990, 725) proposes further steps in helping the practicing physician get to the most useful literature. Journals that clinicians read now have different types of articles mixed together. Haynes identifies the types as scientist to scientist, scientist to practitioner, practitioner to practitioner, and practitioner to scientist. "From the perspective of the clinician, publications from early stages of testing are distracting and potentially dangerous. Serious mistakes can be made in adopting innovations before complete testing" (Hayes 1990, 75). That literature is important, but Haynes feels it can hinder the clinician in getting at the information he or she can use. "Journals that wish to improve biomedical communication can help by choosing the audience they want to serve" (Haynes 1990, 726). The clinician can then reliably pick up a journal knowing that all the articles in it are, for example, covering human clinical trials done with randomized groups. Huth (1989) has written about the underused medical literature. Williamson and others (1989) found the literature inadequately used and proposed rigorous review articles as one way to address the problem.

As medical librarians, we have to see this as an important issue. A few years ago librarians started to talk about quality filtering. This goes back to that idea of finding the "good" articles. We need to play a part in tightening up the "Loose Connections between Peer-Reviewed Clinical Journals and Clinical Practice" (title) that Haynes (1990) explains. Our expertise has developed in finding information on subjects. Our next capability is to separate the wheat from the chaff, since there seems to be enough wheat to eat without having to fill up on the chaff.

MEDICAL (AND MEDICAL LIBRARIAN) IGNORANCE

We see the changes to what is considered the state of the art of medical care. This provides a healthy perspective for you. But what about your patrons—those people who are in the business of caring for sick people? What are their views? They see the new information, too. What is their attitude about the knowledge and beliefs that they apply in their work of diagnosing and treating patients? Are they receptive to new information that contradicts their previously held beliefs and practices? Perhaps the new evidence itself is faulty. It is a difficult proposition to ask people to view what they know as continuously tenuous.

The University of Arizona College of Medicine has been making an interesting attempt to institutionalize this attitude. The medical school has a "Curriculum in Medical Ignorance." "The curriculum consists of seminars and hands-on clinical and laboratory experiences dealing with 'What we know we don't know, what we don't know we don't know, and what we think we know but don't' " (Witte, Kerwin, and Witte 1988, 793). The idea is to make this awareness a part of the future physician's understanding of his or her environment. This stance fits well with the state of medical education. It is understood that there is more medical information today than can be crammed into a medical student's brain in four years. Not only will there be gaps in the state of the field's knowledge, but there will be gaps in the individual's knowledge. Therefore lifelong learning is the best solution. The lesson and attitude must not be put aside after medical school. There is a problem of ''premature closure''—accepting techniques and applying them without the necessary skepticism. ''What these findings imply is that medical educators should beware of residents in less technically developed fields prematurely closing themselves to uncertainties when they have the greatest need to remain open'' (Light 1983, 469).

Be careful not to close your mind either. Actually, librarians new to the field have an advantage in their mindset. Over time, types of questions do become familiar, and it is very easy to become dependent on the sources you already know. MEDLINE is a wonderful tool, for example, and the *AHA Guide to the Health Care Field* is handy. The familiar tools may supply answers, but other ones may be more appropriate for the question at hand. A familiar tool may be relied on too much because that is what you know. To a librarian of the 1990s, every question can be answered by finding the right journal article on MEDLINE (i.e., to a man with a hammer, every problem looks like a nail). This is not a trivial issue. Especially now in the electronic era, you can cultivate sources well beyond these traditional types. Keep your mind open to new sources of information. It sometimes takes a bit of innovation to get the information you need, but what has become available to you is amazing. Be resourceful. Use those resources unknown the previous year. Keep in view the physicians' concern with the overwhelming medical literature. The scope of the electronic resources available to you can be daunting, too.

Besides being on the constant lookout for valuable sources of information, you need to be comfortable in learning new techniques for finding and handling information. You can see that today. The advent of the Gopher for navigating the Internet quickly, in retrospect, gave way to Web browsers. Do not become wedded to a specific means (e.g., the Gopher) of finding the resources any more than you should become attached to the well-worn book or database. Your initiative is needed here more than ever before. What should be the attitude of the reference librarian? You need the drive or desire to answer those questions and an inclination to learn new ways to do it. Both parts are essential. Show patrons that you are intent on finding the answer to their questions. Your internal motivation may be your own curiosity, your sense of satisfaction in solving the problem, your pleasure at learning new things, or even your joy in the hunt. As a health sciences librarian, remember that the eventual goal of the search is the health of the patient. That certainly can supply the motivation. How far are you willing to go in pursuing the answer? Sooner or later you run up against the limits of your experience. In this era of Internet databases, there are seemingly always more places you can check. There is such a thing as diminishing returns. Here is a very important point: If you are comfortable in moving through different interfaces and learning new means of data manipulation during your search, you can go a long way before those diminishing returns are reached. The one thing you cannot now do is be stuck in your own technological development. The easiest thing in the world is to settle on certain ways of doing things or specific databases that you feel comfortable with.

It is still very difficult to use an Internet search tool to find an answer to a specific question (e.g., What is the utilization of radial keratotomy?). Earlier in the chapter we saw that such statistics are often not gathered. On the Internet, you may be able to find "hits" on the topic. However, the lack of authority of much of the information is a formidable problem. As a librarian, you still need to do what you have always done: You need to evaluate the sources. Because the Internet information is moving so quickly, how do you know where the useful information is? You need to keep up with your literature. In this case, your literature may be online newsletters from other librarians or health care personnel. You should monitor the electronic guides to the literature, so to speak. It is now an important part of your job to know what is reliable and useful on the Internet, and you should develop a way to update yourself continuously. When the questions come in from your patrons, the wealth of sources at your command can be great. Can all this really be at your command? You cannot really be expected to know all there is to know. What is expected of you? The same thing that has always been expected of reference librarians, namely, the ability and initiative to know how to go about finding the information. Twenty years ago we began going beyond our four walls for information on electronic networks. Now we go far beyond our well-organized bibliographic networks of MEDLINE and the Online Computer Library Center (OCLC).

GETTING ON THE ELECTRONIC REFERENCE TRAIL

Here is one example of how you and your clientele might use these resources. The Human Genome Project (Keleher 1993) is big science. Its goals include identifying all the genes in a human being (100,000?), analyzing each gene to determine its structure, linking the gene with its function, understanding the mechanisms of genetic diseases, and then finding a way to cure or prevent the diseases. This is leading us to a dramatic change in how medicine is practiced. When we see that news story on how a gene has been linked to Alzheimer's or alcoholism, for instance, we can now go to the specific data behind the report. Previously, the raw data just resided in the laboratory notebooks and was unavailable to most. Of course, we have always seen the evidence of progress with the accumulation of journal articles in the field. We can find a lot of literature on the Human Genome Project, too, and at several levels—for the public, for the biomedical researcher, and for the practicing physician. Not to belittle the journal article, a more dynamic tool is needed here. One of those dynamic tools is GenBank (Woodsmall and Benson 1993). Scientists store their findings about gene sequences and protein sequences in GenBank. Scientists and physicians search GenBank and other repositories. Dr. Crozier, for example, is investigating a specific gene and would like to see any sequencing done on it. He can search by the name or position of the gene on the chromosome. In contrast, Dr. Hodge has found a sequence in the laboratory and wants to see if that sequence matches anything identified already. One reason this information is helpful is that sequences found to be similar in structure may also be similar in function (Altschul et al. 1990). Such findings are certainly one of the goals of the project, which is attempting to map genes to their functions. He can send a specifically designed e-mail message through the Basic Local Alignment Search Tool (BLAST) software with the amino acid, nucleotide, or protein sequence he found. In this way the findings and data can be checked by anyone with access to GenBank. There is no charge, and it is available on the Internet. Give Westheimer a break (Crampon 1988). You can show your patrons how to get started on this and on many paths to information. Chapter 6 provides a sampling of the computer applications useful to you and your clientele.

REFERENCE LIBRARIAN AS INSTRUCTOR

We want it to be easy to find information. The "we" in this case is inclusive: end users, information producers, and librarians, too. Look what happened with MEDLINE. Making it simple and accessible to use on CD-ROM has greatly expanded its use by our patrons. Tools are being developed to find meaningful information on the World Wide Web more successfully. Now libraries are often called upon to help find useful Internet databases. Web browsers are improving. Perhaps that role of Internet guide will decline as our role as MEDLINE intermediaries has declined. What, then, for us? If we are not called upon as intermediaries, as guides to the information, what will be the role for the reference librarian? It may be naive to think that our help will no longer be needed in finding information. However, our main mission may shift to teaching people how to find their own information. This is not a radical change. We have always been doing some of this. Moving beyond the books and journals is not new to medical librarians. Health sciences libraries regard themselves as trailblazers in the electronic era (MEDLINE being an early electronic database). Audiovisual materials became an important part of collections and services in many hospital and medical school libraries. Now we see exciting developments that combine computerization and audiovisuals. A 1986 long-range plan encouraged NLM "to consider building and disseminating medical image libraries much the same way it acquires, indexes, and provides access to the biomedical literature" (National Library Medicine 1995c). This led to the Visible Human Project. Indeed, there are many opportunities for medical libraries and medical librarians.

Physicians have been challenged to master the means of lifelong learning (Association of American Medical Colleges 1984). This is the natural role for us. Here is one application. For a number of years now physicians and others have had the opportunity and often the inclination to gather information that they have found useful and store it in their own databases. Several programs designed to store bibliographic information on a personal computer are available (e.g., Reference Manager, Pro-Cite, EndNote). Physicians could use our guidance in starting and using these programs. We can explain and demonstrate a number of issues that they may want to address in building their database. Consider the following:

1. How will they be retrieving information from their file (e.g., by author, by subject, by Boolean combinations)?
2. How will they select their subject headings?
3. Will they be using a standardized list of headings or making up their own?
4. How will they assign headings to the articles in their database?
5. Will they be downloading information from other databases and/or keying in the data?
6. How will they be arranging the physical collection (reprints, etc.): classified, alphabetical, chronological?
7. What will they be doing about updating their file and weeding out the obsolete information?
8. What will be in their collection? just articles? books? technical reports? slides?
9. With their needs, what software would be best for them?

This is an obvious area that calls upon our teaching expertise. It is tied very closely to the things we have always done in organizing our collection and our need for information retrieval. Much of the information available today is not bibliographic. However, our ideas in organization and retrieval will be helpful in teaching others to find their own information. There is a demand for this expertise. Librarians are not the only people who may wish to fill that role. If we limit ourselves to the bibliographic information, others will take over from us.

6

Computerization of Biomedical Information

INTRODUCTION

You might say that we are entering a golden age of medical information. Even better than that, in the spirit of John Shaw Billings and Lister Hill (his encouragement comes in Chapter 7), it is a golden age of access to medical information. This chapter focuses on information that our clientele can and do use now. They access it from their preferred sites—their office or their lab or their home or their patient's bedside. This has been a goal or vision or dream of librarians for some time. The 1980s witnessed the initiation of a formal plan, IAIMS (Integrated Academic [or Advanced] Information Management System), intended to reach toward that goal. In the 1990s IAIMS has been overshadowed and overtaken by the universal access provided by the Internet. We will look at a sampling of electronic medical resources available via the Internet and also resources residing in your library. Organizing and searching sources under your control in the library is one thing, but it does get harder once you have moved beyond the four walls. You will need to

1. know what is "out there"
2. evaluate what is "out there"
3. "organize" what is "out there"

This brief list contained an unseemly number of terms in quotation marks. Why is this presented here with such a lack of precision? The Internet is intimidating.

We do not obtain information in the same way we did before. What we need is a way to view or approach the world of electronic information so that we can with some confidence find reliable and pertinent data when we need it.

HOW TO FIND ELECTRONIC INFORMATION

In the past we have analyzed and indexed and cataloged biomedical publications. Can we really do that with electronic resources residing at thousands of sites spread throughout the world, with new ones appearing and others disappearing each day? There are two general strategies we can use to go about handling biomedical information on the Internet.

1. *Use our traditional model.* Rely on guides to the electronic literature, so to speak. Librarians and others have been evaluating medical sources on the Internet and grading them on utility, accuracy, currency, authority, and so on. They may be slotted into different categories, as we slotted the print reference tools we examined in Chapter 5. We could learn the useful electronic sources in the same way you have learned about key books on internal medicine, a sort of dynamic, electronic Brandon list.

2. *Use smart searching systems.* Rely on searching algorithms that search across databanks with ever more powerful relevancy-weighting systems. We saw the beginnings of that at the end of Chapter 3 with WIN (Westlaw Is Natural) and WAIS. It likely will be impractical to organize the electronic sources in the way we have cataloged books or even the way NLM has indexed journal articles. Instead of doing the work of organizing and categorizing beforehand, we can do it afterward at the searching stage. This has fundamental implications on how we go about our job. Earlier we discussed something of the pros and cons of this. Taking the effort to use a controlled vocabulary, such as MeSH, at the input end saves time on the searching end. Compare searching those databases with their indexing and controlled vocabulary with the ones that are searchable by free text only. We have seen that simple free text searching is generally inadequate even for the bibliographic databases. For the Internet and its full-text files, we definitely need something more powerful. That is where those smart searching systems come in.

This smart searching path to information has an allure to it for this era. As we have seen, physicians in the *GPEP Report* (Association of American Medical Colleges 1984) have been urged to master the means of lifelong learning. In practice, this means finding solutions to a problem when that problem comes up. Memorizing old solutions learned in medical school or gathered from a medical textbook will not be adequate. First, it will be impossible to memorize enough. Second, memorization does not keep the physician up to date. Knowing how to find information is the key. To a degree, physicians are urged to acquire some of the skills that librarians have always used. This orientation fits in with an outlook we have heard about before in the library in collection development: "just in time" instead of "just in case." Can we in the library afford to buy materials for our clientele in the belief that they will probably want them—to have them just in case they ask for them? Or do we need to be able to find and obtain information and documents at the time of demand? This service is at the heart of the idea of the virtual library. If we can obtain and deliver information at the point of demand, what is the need for ownership of a collection? Is there a need for a librarian if there is no library? If you view librarianship as a service as opposed to stewardship over a warehouse, there could be a much greater role for librarians in the future than in the past.

Right now there is no need to make that choice between the traditional methods of organizing applied to electronic resources and the new kind of searching. We can use them both if the smart searching system is smart enough. There is an important question that must be asked, however. With the smart systems, can we factor in measurements of quality of the information or database into the algorithm? Can those measurements be factored in and yield results that we trust? For now, anyway, the searching system may not be sufficient. Fortunately, there is definitely a demand for better and better searching systems on the Internet, and this demand goes well beyond the librarians. We should be able to adopt some of these innovations. Before a physician can call up the information from the bedside or a researcher can call it up from the laboratory bench or a student can call it up from the classroom, the library, the hospital, and so on, the information needs to be evaluated. Just because data may be easily available does not imply they are useful. Significant steps need to have been taken before our patrons can easily and confidently make that "call up." First, a system must be constructed with linkages to the varied computerized sources within the institution and beyond. Second, the data itself must be of high quality and pertinent to the need. Third, the user (physician, researcher, nurse, etc.) must be able to request and satisfactorily retrieve information with his or her own terminology. Having to learn an arcane set of commands and formal vocabulary will inhibit the utility of the system.

How do we get there? We are making real progress. This chapter presents some initiatives that health sciences libraries are joining, planning, and implementing. Although the few sources covered here are important, even more than those covered in Chapter 5, they represent but a tiny portion of what is "out there."

INTEGRATION OF INFORMATION: IAIMS

NLM initiated the grant program for IAIMS in 1982. Integrating the diverse sources of biomedical information in an academic health center and a hospital was a key motivation for IAIMS (Matheson and Cooper 1982). Each system in the institution had been built for its own use and was independent of the others. On a smaller scale, libraries have done this, too. In the library, it is certainly convenient to have the online catalog integrated with the circulation system and with the acquisitions system and with the serials system. In IAIMS, the online catalog may be accessed from the same menu as molecular biology databases or the hospital's surgery scheduling. ''Yesterday's information seeker had to rely on a personal arsenal of telephone numbers, access codes, log-in procedures, and searching strategies. Because of IAIMS, today's information seeker is guided through the network and navigates from database to database and system to system in a seamless fashion. A user's effort is spent in using the information, not looking for it'' (Broering 1993, 22). Another motivation for the IAIMS initiative was to involve the library in information gathering and dissemination beyond our bibliographic environment. People need and will use information from other sources. Librarians should be involved for two reasons. We know about information retrieval, so there is a contribution we can make. The other reason is this: We do not want to be left behind holding the bound volumes while the role of information service moves on to others. The original IAIMS projects have now had several years of planning and development (Lorenzi 1992). The three programs covered below are implementing the common goals of IAIMS with their own directions: one-stop shopping; linkage of the scholarly and the clinical; and hypertext.

The Georgetown University Medical Center's Dahlgren Memorial Library has developed a Knowledge Network (Broering 1993) that provides users one place to go for their information needs. It contains databases separated into modules: bibliographic, information, diagnostic, and research. The bibliographic module covers citations to books and journal articles. The information module includes full-text databases on drugs, poisons, and cancer. The diagnostic systems are interactive programs intended for practitioners and students to assist them in determining probable diagnoses of illnesses of patients. The research databases include gene sequence information and project-funding opportunities. Educational software and incorporation of a patient care information system from the hospital side are additional pieces. Workstations for the practitioner, student, researcher, and faculty have all had to be designed and connected. The linking of diverse systems—the hardware, the software, and the communications—has not been a trivial matter for the IAIMS projects. However, this has had to be done. The network has to be convenient for the user if it is to be used. Admittedly, the library has not been alone in the construction of IAIMS. It has involved the expertise, cooperation, and resources of the whole institution—the academic health centers with the hospital.

The IAIMS project at the Columbia-Presbyterian Medical Center has been successful in linking the clinical information systems (Roderer and Clayton 1992). The broad categories in this network are scholarly information systems, clinical decision making, and clinical results reporting. The scholarly information includes MEDLINE, an online catalog, as well as electronic textbooks. The clinical decision making has medical records, surgery scheduling, and DRG coding information. The clinical results have patient data from the laboratory, pathology, and radiology. In addition to the technical problems of merging these diverse systems, matters of access to patient data and privacy have to be understood and incorporated into the system.

A hypertext concept has been used by the Baylor College of Medicine to develop what it calls the Virtual Notebook System (VNS). The biomedical researchers at Baylor are the main community for which this system is intended. ''It is a distributed, multimedia hypertext system that transcends many limitations of pencil and paper. Users of the VNS share work with one another through notebooks that any number of group members may own. . . . [I]t may consist of text and images captured from any other window or program on the user's display'' (Gorry 1992, 249–250). The Neuroscience Division may, for example, set up a link to a databank of neuroanatomy images or molecular biology sequences. The connection remains for the next time that researcher or another researcher opens the VNS. The numbers and types of links will depend on the individual needs of the person or group involved with the research.

INTEGRATION OF INFORMATION: THE INTERNET

The protocols of Internet communication and capabilities of client-server systems are well beyond the capabilities of this author and therefore the range of this book. However, during the ten years that IAIMS architectures have been under construction in a few dozen academic health sciences centers, a revolution in the linkage of computers has taken place. The Internet has come to the people. Millions of people—including researchers, physicians, nurses, students, and librarians—connect to databanks around the world every day. In a short amount of time this has become routine. It has become routine partly because institutions have set up first Gophers and then Web home pages to enable users to move through the Internet with menus. Each menu choice or link provides more choices and databanks. In a way, the IAIMS links to a handful of sources, discussed earlier, seem somewhat meager. However, it should be noted that the menus in the IAIMS in-house selections also feature links to outside the institution through the Internet.

A natural link for health sciences libraries is to the National Institutes of Health (NIH). The NIH home page or Gopher provides the link to several resources of use to clinicians and researchers. Let's take a closer look first at one clinical tool noted for its high quality and usefulness, CancerNet. To get there through the World Wide Web, use a Web browser such as Netscape to connect to the Uniform Resource Locator (URL) for the NIH.

http://www.nih.gov

You are greeted with the following menu:

Welcome to the National Institutes of Health

Welcome to NIH

News & Events
Health Information
Grants & Contracts
Scientific Resources
Institutes & Offices

To get to CancerNet, select Health Information. Your choices there also include AIDS Related Information; NIH Consensus Development Program; HSTAT (Health Services/Technology Assessment Text); and NIH Information Index. Selecting the NIH Gopher CancerNet Menu retrieves

Complete CancerNet Contents List
PDQ Information (Current Clinical Cancer Information)
CancerNet News
Publications
Fact Sheets from the NCI
Monthly Update Information
Search CancerNet Database
CANCERLIT Citations and Abstracts

Select PDQ Information and retrieve this menu from the Physician Data Query:

PDQ Treatment Statements for Physicians
PDQ Treatment Statements for Patients
PDQ Supportive Care Statements
PDQ Screening/Prevention Statements
PDQ Drug Information Statements
Other PDQ Information

The PDQ statements are especially valuable because they are reviewed so frequently (monthly) and are overseen by a board of experts in the field. This finally addresses successfully one of the big problems in medical information. It serves to evaluate new information for clinicians so they can use it with patients they are treating now. Current information useful for treating patients—that is exactly what we have been wanting to find. As we move beyond our peer-reviewed biomedical journals, mechanisms need to be set up to assist us in finding reliable and useful information from sources that are not so familiar to us. CancerNet is an Internet system that has been praised for meeting the needs of accessibility, reliability, usefulness, and timeliness (Hancock 1994). This information system from the National Cancer Institute can be utilized by Internet connections with Telnet and Gopher as well as via e-mail and fax. One part of CancerNet consists of discussions of treatment for different types of cancers. Each of these state-of-the-art recommendations is available at two levels: one for the physician and another one written at a level understandable by patients, families, and consumers.The PDQ Treatment Statements for Physicians have the following: prognosis, cellular classification, stage information, treatment option overview, and treatment options for specific stages. The PDQ Treatment Statements for Patients have these: overview of PDQ, which describes PDQ and how to use it; description of that cancer; stage explanation; treatment option overview; treatment by stage; and information on where to go to learn more.

Also on CancerNet are full-text fact sheets from the National Cancer Institute as well as citations and abstracts of the most recent six months of CANCERLIT, a MEDLARS database that you would otherwise need an account and password to search. CancerNet right now does not include an important part of PDQ—the clinical trials protocols. The protocols section describes ongoing clinical research programs and also provides eligibility information for cancer patients interested in joining those studies. As part of the research, the patients could receive treatments of drugs or techniques still under investigation. To find this information now, use the PDQ file on the MEDLARS online searching system. Would not the next step for medical information be to have medical organizations, perhaps other divisions of NIH or professional groups such as the American Board of Medical Specialties, devise their own Nets (e.g., HeartNet or DiabetesNet or BackNet)? This type of activity is taking place, but without coordination. Some government agencies have been quick to provide Internet information, whereas others have lagged behind. CancerNet provides a model.

THE INTERNET AS A RESEARCH TOOL: MOLECULAR BIOLOGY

Whether you have taken a hypertext route or a Gopher route or made a direct Telnet connection, there is that question of quality of the information. What happens to the serials literature with the coming of electronic journals? The issue of editorial overview and peer reviewing is always brought up. Will changing the traditional format from paper to electronic mean that we forego the gatekeeping functions of editors and referees? In our utilization of data on the Internet, we go far beyond "electronic journals." The question that we as consumers of information and as organizers of information (librarians) have to address is the quality of the data that we are connecting to and retrieving. For instance, it may not be sufficient to help molecular biologists link to GenBank. We should find out how information gets into GenBank. Is most of the sequence information derived from the journal literature? Is other data submitted and accepted without having been published and, therefore, without having the legitimacy that that implies? You can continue to offer a "collection development" service by looking for what is useful for your clientele and finding evaluations of the databanks. Typically, we will not have the expertise to evaluate all data ourselves, but we can consult with our patrons. They are experts in the subject fields and will be using the data. Let us take molecular biology as an example.

Several times in this book molecular biology databanks have been mentioned. Molecular biology is the very symbol of basic research biology. At the same time, the importance of providing mature, trustworthy information to the clinician has been emphasized, and techniques for finding it have been suggested. The popular press as well as the biomedical literature tells us that the genetic revolution is at hand. Take a look at the cover stories that appeared in consecutive months: in *Newsweek*, ''The Hunt for the Breast Cancer Gene'' (Cowley 1993), and in *Time*, ''Genetics: The Future Is Now'' (Elmer-DeWitt 1994). Physicians will be able to diagnose diseases on the basis of the composition of the gene and will be able to use gene therapy to correct the condition. Health sciences librarians need to acquire some background information here to see what is going on around them. The following is an extremely modest primer on key areas from the research to patient care.

The description in 1953 by James Watson and Francis Crick of the structure of deoxyribonucleic acid (DNA) initiated the current era. Often characterized as the molecule that provides the ''blueprint'' for life—the directions for how we are constructed (Rosenthal 1994)—DNA provides the instructions on how to make proteins. These proteins form the color of our eyes and the structure of hemoglobin in our red blood cells. Proteins are the enzymes that instruct our bodies how to utilize sugar. In other words, the correct workings of our bodies are dependent on the instructions from DNA. This genetic material is in every cell in the body and, in humans, is carried within 23 pairs of chromosomes. It is estimated that about 100,000 genes are parcelled out in those 23 chromosomes. Each gene, it is thought, can be linked to a specific protein or an individual function in the body. In some cases a single gene does not have the full instructions for a function, but in other cases it does. In order to understand the specific instructions, genes must be identified.

—We need to find where they are on the chromosome and identify what trait in our bodies they control.

—Beyond that, we need to see of what the gene itself is constructed. For basic biology, we want to see its structure so that we can gain an understanding of how our bodies work.

—For medicine, we need to see how our bodies are supposed to function in order to correct malfunctions (e.g., when the patient has diabetes or cystic fibrosis).

—For treatment, we want to find techniques to use in order to alter or override defective genes (i.e., gene therapy).

The Human Genome Project's goal is to identify and characterize all 100,000 genes in the human body. Because certain other organisms have fewer genes than humans do and some genes in those animals seem to give instructions analogous to ones in humans, part of the project includes looking for what are termed homologies. Impressive databanks are acting as registries of information where researchers can deposit their findings (Martin, Primich, and Riley 1994). These databanks represent steps along the way of the goal of the Human Genome Project. The Genome Data Base (GDB) has as one of its missions the location of the genes on the chromosomes. Because a gene cannot be isolated by sight, techniques have been and are being developed to identify them. These developing techniques are part of the GDB. The GDB and the Online Mendelian Inheritance in Man (OMIM) databases are located at the Johns Hopkins University School of Medicine. The latter contains the clinical data on genetic diseases with information on genetic linkage.

Going down another level from the specific gene and its location and the diseases associated with its malfunction is the structure of the gene itself. What is each gene made up of? GenBank acts as a repository of this information. Undeniably, molecular genetics is a complicated subject, but familiarity with some of the concepts and terms will go a long way in helping you assist your patrons in their search for information. The genetic material of the gene is deoxyribonucleic acid. It is composed of nucleic acids, which are composed of nucleotides. Nucleotides contain sugars, phosphates, and bases. The bases are what we want to focus on. The four bases are adenine (a), thymine (t), guanine (g), and cytosine (c), and they form base pairs: adenine goes with thymine and guanine goes with cytosine. The big picture is that DNA codes for proteins and more specifically for enzymes, and we want to find the codes. The code is arranged this way: The message from sets of three bases is called the codon. Each of these encodes for an amino acid. The twenty standard amino acids are the building blocks of the proteins. Therefore, the sequence of the material in DNA parallels the sequence of material of the proteins. A clearly written, highly recommended, and interestingly illustrated book to begin your investigation is *The Cartoon Guide to Genetics*, and here is an irreverent, representative passage: "The subunits of protein molecules are amino acids, which are not named after Idi Amin, the former dictator of Uganda" (Gonick and Wheelis 1991, 108).

In GenBank, you will see arrangements of *a* and *t* and *c* and *g*, representing sequences of nucleotides. Other databanks have the sequences of proteins and still other databanks include the sequences of the genomes of other organisms. Now let's look at GenBank. One way to get to it is the same route you took to use CancerNet. Instead of opening the "Health Information" menu item, use "Scientific Resources." Another path to GenBank is to directly open a location on the World Wide Web, http://www.ncbi.nlm.nih.gov. Once there, you may search in various ways. Your patron may have discovered a sequence in the lab and wants to match it against the database. He or she could enter the *a*'s and *t*'s and *c*'s and *g*'s with the BLAST software (Altschul et al. 1990) for statistical comparisons against the sequences already in GenBank. It would be difficult to imagine that this searching could be done as efficiently any other way than via the Internet.

Perhaps your patron wants to use GenBank to see research on a disease (e.g.,

Alzheimer's disease). To find ''hits'' on Alzheimer's in humans, one way to search is ''alzheimer and sapiens.'' (GenBank does take Boolean operators.) The first ''hit'' out of 105 is ''Human germline immunoglobulin heavy chain variable region (VH-III family) for anti-B-amyloid autoantibodies in Alzheimer's disease.'' This is a record taken from a journal article in *Clinical Immunology and Immunopathology* in 1995 and includes a MEDLINE accession number, too. This entry for Alzheimer's shows information on chromosome 14 and the sequence of 478 bases is given, starting with

gactgcacac agagaactca cca . . .

In order to bring this information from biological research to clinical medicine, it needs to prove useful in diagnosing genetic disorders and providing therapies. ''The possibility of gene therapy was first discussed in the late 1960s and early 1970s, after it had been demonstrated that mammalian cells could take up and express exogenous DNA'' (Levine and Friedmann 1993, 1167). This means it is possible to insert the coding material into the cell in order to remedy a faulty mechanism of protein production. Techniques using viruses and other means are being experimented with now to do just that. One of these is with cystic fibrosis.

> Cystic fibrosis is one of the most common genetic diseases caused by a single genetic defect. The responsible gene, termed CFTR, is a transmembrane protein that has the properties of a chloride transporter. Because of the high prevalence of CF and the relative ineffectiveness of drug therapy at present, approaches to gene therapy are being pursued intensively. (Levine and Friedmann 1993, 1173)

Will molecular genetics transform the practice of medicine? ''The emphasis in medical research has slowly shifted from the study of disease at the level of patients or their diseased organs to the study of their cells and molecules. Although major scientific achievements do not always have practical benefits for many years, we already know enough about the potential value of molecular biology to predict that the medical sciences are moving into their most exciting and productive period'' (Weatherall 1995, 228). With newspapers reporting every week on the discovery of another gene linked to a disease, this expectation is becoming widely held.

FINDING RESEARCH FUNDING ON THE INTERNET

Patient care, research, and money—these are three concerns of your patrons. In order for your clientele to conduct their research, they need funds. The NIH has been a main source of funding, and some paper-based publications do alert investigators to funding opportunities. Let's look at researchers' access to this information now that it has migrated to an electronic form. Go back once again to the NIH Gopher and select the item "Grants and Research Information." Select "NIH Guide to Grants and Contracts." Here are announcements of the availability of funds for medical research. You can scan "Requests for Applications" or "Requests for Proposals," or you can search the database with keywords (e.g., "cardiovascular"). Another way to look at funding is identifying research that has already been awarded to institutions. Computer Retrieval of Information on Scientific Projects (CRISP) has that information. This is searchable, too, and you can find what has been awarded by subject or institution or by names of investigators. These databases from NIH are free. There are, however, other electronic repositories of funding information that your users may wish to have access to. One of these is Sponsored Programs Information Network (SPIN). This system has both federal funders and nonfederal funders in it. It is not free but may be subscribed to and operated by the office of research administration at your institution.

THE TERMINOLOGY ISSUE

Even while examining the new fields in biology and the coming sophisticated search tools, one of the oldest issues in librarianship needs to be looked at again. That has to do with vocabulary control. To do effective searching of the literature, librarians and patrons have had to use the subject headings and thesauruses used to catalog books and index articles. To make these IAIMS projects or virtual information systems effective, the barrier of our rigid terminology systems has to be removed. The UMLS (Unified Medical Language System) was noted in Chapter 3. One goal is to enable physicians and other users of Grateful Med to use their own terms and expressions and still search MEDLINE effectively. For example, a physician could enter "kidney stone" or "renal calculi" or "kidney calculi" or "kidney disease," and so on, and receive the appropriate information. Not a trivial matter, this development with the searching of MEDLINE is not difficult to visualize. It is when we go beyond our comfortable borders and happen upon the numerous other computerized sources of information that health care professionals use and will use in the future and that are connected by the Internet do we see the scope of the difficulties our terminology may cause us. There are other initiatives, too. In Europe, the Generalized Architecture for Languages, Encyclopedias, and Nomenclatures (GALEN) in medicine is analogous to the activities of the UMLS (Rada et al. 1992). Cognitive science, computer science, linguistics, and psychology all have a hand in studying natural language processing and will lead us to more natural ways of searching for all kinds of information.

MEDICAL INFORMATICS

Shortliffe and Perreault's (1990) book title gives the general definition of "medical informatics": *Medical Informatics: Computer Applications in Health*

Care. More specifically, "medical informatics is the field concerned with the cognitive, information processing, and communication tasks of medical practice, education, and research, including the information science and technology to support these tasks" (Greenes and Shortliffe 1990, 1115). Information processing, medical practice, and information science—this sounds like something within the scope and interests of health sciences libraries. Medical informatics, as demonstrated by these broad definitions, encompasses many applications. Two of them are the (1) computerized patient record and (2) medical decision support systems.

The medical record of the patient is analogous to the laboratory notebook. The laboratory notebook often has the fullest account of the research project but is available only to those working on the project. It is not in the open literature but does contain important data. The patient's medical record is also not publicly available. This is partly due to matters of privacy. Separating the clinical information on the course of the diseases and the treatments from the identity of the patient will enable the wider use of the data while protecting the individual patients. The patient's chart is also often still handwritten, not systematic, and without a controlled terminology. Were the information about the patient computerized in a standardized form, and detailed with a clinical, uniform vocabulary, there would be benefits both for that individual patient and patients at large. For an individual patient, the data could be connected to an expert system that has a codification of such things as dangerous drug interactions and abnormal readings of laboratory tests. Then if a drug were prescribed that would yield adverse reactions in that patient, a signal would appear from the computer system warning against it. Or, using CancerNet, the latest treatment protocols for specific cancers could be linked into the information system of the patient. Better care should result for the patient with these knowledge bases built into the system. For purposes of research, the treatments and conditions of many people could be compiled to get information about successful and unsuccessful interventions. Data could be gathered for short-term therapies of acute conditions and also to see comparative health outcomes of patients over many years. This would provide a wealth of epidemiological information. Proponents also point to advantages in administrative and economic aspects. When people move or change health care providers, the records are more easily available and reimbursement information is obtained more quickly. The Institute of Medicine's (Dick and Steen 1991) report on the computer-based patient record provided the impetus for the Computer-based Patient Record Institute. This action reflects the fact that the move from the traditional paper-based system will not come easily and quickly. Also, the computerization of the data will not be sufficient to reach the goals. "Without a more structured method of data collection using a standard controlled vocabulary, it will be impossible to make rational decisions about which treatments are cost-effective and how patient outcomes are affected by our clinical decisions" (Barnett, Jenders, and Chueh 1993, 1047). Here is our terminology issue again.

Medical decision support systems are other programs that fall within medical informatics. The MedIndEx project was discussed in Chapter 3 as a way to assist indexers of journal articles by programming the rules and guides into a "smart" computer system. This knowledge base that interacts with the human indexer gives the novice a context-sensitive application of the rules and enables an expert level of indexing. "Both of these systems [Quick Medical Reference and Iliad] operate in a textbook mode for reading the knowledge base, a consultation mode for generating advice on patient work-ups, and a simulation mode where students attempt to reach a diagnosis on a simulated patient by ordering tests" (Broering 1993, 24). A real objective is to construct an expert system that truly reflects the knowledge and know-how of a human expert. Moving from the use of medical students in learning to clinicians in treating patients with state-of-the-art information would represent impressive improvements in these systems. Some of the answers may come with advances in artificial intelligence and/or neural networks research. Librarians need to keep up-to-date in the development of medical software. We can follow their progress with software reviews as we always did for books with book reviews. See, for example, "Performance of Four Computer-Based Diagnostic Systems" (Berner et al. 1994).

Medical informatics demands the collaborative efforts of information science and medicine. Organizations form, journals start, and meetings are held (e.g., American Medical Informatics Association, *International Journal of Biomedical Computing*, and Symposium on Computer Applications in Medical Care). There is a section of the MLA on medical informatics. The *Medical Reference Service Quarterly* includes a column entitled "Medical Informatics."

ELECTRONIC FULL-TEXT WITH MULTIMEDIA

Journals and books are appearing in a variety of electronic formats. For journals, a great part of the attraction is speed and even convenience. If a researcher can search MEDLINE and click on a citation and pull up the full text of the article, that certainly beats requesting it via interlibrary loan or even looking for it in the stacks of the local library. Several varieties of electronic journals are available: current titles are now produced also on CD-ROM; titles, mostly individual articles, are scanned and stored in remote computers for purchase on demand; and newly created journals are designed only for electronic delivery. Although medical libraries have been asking this question for a number of years, how long can we keep weathering 10% and 20% price increases for our serials? Is the answer in the electronic journal and the acquisition of this specialized information article by article?

The trusted and well-used core textbooks of medicine are now being produced with multimedia capabilities. The CD-ROM version can offer moving pictures and sounds (e.g., see and hear the beating of the heart). No longer does a student or teacher need to find a separate videocassette or set of slides or audiocassette. The CD-ROM can have sounds and pictures and even animation right along with the text. This sounds like a very attractive solution to make learning and teaching more convenient. The students and teachers will be spending their time learning instead of looking for information. When does all this happen? It is happening now. The cost factor goes in the right direction. Computer processing costs less and less; information processing with paper costs more and more. Where does that leave the discussions in previous chapters on the biomedical journal and the core textbooks? Regardless of form, students and practitioners will still need to depend on information that has gone through critical evaluation. Either in the traditional way or in new ways of reviewing or editing, that function will be needed.

TELEMEDICINE

Technology and cost—these are driving factors in today's health care. Normally, technology is thought of as a key factor in the rising cost of health care. Advances in radiology, for example, with magnetic resonance imaging or positron electron tomography provide better diagnostic information than the simple x-ray. The equipment is also more costly. Can technology be put to use in telemedicine to provide both improved care and lower cost? The conclusive answer may not quite be at hand, but here is the idea. Medical students are trained in medical centers, which include the most advanced technology, expertise, and knowledge in the world. Many then go off to practice in rural areas. Because it would not pay to have all the experts move to the rural areas—there would not be enough demand—the primary care physician faces a problem. Can he or she diagnose or treat the disease, or should he or she recommend that the patient travel to the medical center? What the physician in the rural community needs is the expertise of the medical center. Telemedicine offers this. With high-capacity digital lines, real-time two-way communication is becoming a reality. With teleradiology, for example, the experts back at the medical center and the clinician with the patient can look at the images at the same time. The patient is rewarded with more expert care, and the clinician gains information. Telemedicine is mostly still in its experimental stage, but some would forecast the day that the digital connection through cable in your home will provide what Dr. Jay Sanders calls the "electronic house call" (Carlson 1994). Hookups such as an electronic stethoscope will make it possible to monitor chronically ill patients without trips to the doctor's office or hospital. We have seen the possibilities of electronic information sources and the virtual library. What about the virtual hospital?

THE VIRTUAL HOSPITAL AND THE INTERACTIVE PATIENT

Plenty of sites from medical centers and elsewhere have organized medical information on the Internet. Many of them are set up to provide their users with links to Internet sites of interest. Many also provide the resource itself—the site others link to. Here are two examples that have interesting names and seem to be right up our alley:

The Virtual Hospital (URL—http://indy.radiology.uiowa.edu)
The Interactive Patient (URL—http://musom.marshall.edu)

With experience you will find the Internet locations of use for your patrons and link them to your library's or institution's home page. When you are looking for specific information to answer a question or in general for good sources to link, you can consult an Internet bibliography. Gary Malet and Lee Hancock have been compiling lists of medical resources on the Internet since "the early days." Of course, that was not that many years ago, but they were pioneers. Look on the Web for

Medical Matrix—Guide to Internet Clinical Medical Resources
(http://www.kumc.edu:80/mmatrix)

InterCat (http://www.oclc.org:6990) is a project begun in 1995 by OCLC to catalog Internet resources. The records are in MARC format and are designed to be included in a library's online catalog. A key field in the record is for the electronic access point (e.g., URL). Will the library's process of organization, cataloging, be useful for information retrieval on the Internet (Flannery 1995)?

The goal of health sciences information is to make these rich databanks available for widespread use. The revolution has to come into the physician's office. Remember again the *GPEP Report* (Association of American Medical Colleges 1984). When that was written ten years ago, a large part of that mastery could have been achieved with the medical literature. The physician would develop a systematic means of reading the medical literature and, probably, search MEDLINE. In the middle of the 1990s that is no longer sufficient. The physician now, at least, must connect to and use the Internet (Glowniak and Bushway 1994).

The coverage of computerization of biomedical information offered in this chapter is inadequate. It is not even the tip of the iceberg. It is not even the ice chips sitting on top of the iceberg. (Sorry about the hyperbole.) You know the fast pace of biomedicine. This leads us to how you as the health sciences librarian should keep up to date and develop the habits of lifelong learning. This and other matters are the subjects of Chapter 7.

7

The Habitat of the Health Sciences Librarian

INTRODUCTION

Health sciences librarians are found in hospitals, medical schools, schools for other health care professionals, biomedical research organizations, companies, medical associations and societies, and more. As you look at what we do and where we work, you notice an omission from the chapters so far. There have been discussions about the biomedical literature, how to find information, what materials to buy, the attributes of computerized systems, how to deliver services, and innovations in biomedical computing. However, a lot was just assumed. Along the way, it was assumed that you had an overall plan for your library to deliver the services. You have investigated your users' needs. In response, you have investigated appropriate technologies, made agreements for the equipment and services, arranged for the physical space of a library, and obtained training for yourself and your staff. To deliver meaningful service, you also need to establish working relations with individuals and groups both within and outside your institution. You need that information both to understand your users' needs and to know where to go to find solutions to their information problems. The search for information is not possible without the tools, and the delivery of services is not effective without knowledge of your environment. This is not a one-time learning experience. You will need to evaluate, add to, and change what you do and how you do it on an ongoing basis. Learn all you can about the environment in which you work and the people you work with.

Hospital libraries comprise the largest group of health sciences libraries—2,167 in the latest comprehensive survey (American Hospital Association 1991). The economic climate is of vital interest to the hospital librarian, a special librarian. Special libraries are not taken as a given or viewed as "public goods" the way public libraries or college libraries are regarded. When economic constraints have been placed on an organization, the special library is not the last place an administration has looked to make cuts. The hospital has been going through dramatic changes in its role. The status quo has not been an option. A special library needs to demonstrate actively and innovatively the advantages it gives an organization. If it does not, the library may not only see its budget cut, it may be eliminated. We know that the information we provide is indispensable and even cost-effective to the functions of health care. However, your confidence in the role of the library is not enough. Make sure your patrons and administrators understand what you do and how it helps them. Our susceptibility to closing is one very good reason that we need to understand the economics of health care. A healthful habitat for the library is dependent on our knowledge of the economic environment, macro and micro.

MACROECONOMICS OF HEALTH CARE

There are many fine books covering library management. Much of that information applies to health sciences libraries and does not need to be repeated here. Also, there are a ton of books published in the 1990s on the economics of health care, so that should not be examined in depth in this chapter either. Therefore, the following presents just a sketch of the economic environment in which we, especially hospital librarians, work. The dollar figures and percentages associated with health care have become familiar in the last few years—a trillion dollars and 14% of GNP. Health care is big business, and its considerable portion of the total economy is why the cost of health care is so often a topic of discussion. We need some historical context. Kronenfeld and Whicker's (1984) figures show the trend.

National Health Expenditures (Amount and Percentage of GNP):

1950—$12.7 billion—4.4%
1980—$247.2 billion—9.4% (p. 4)

Percentage of National Health Expenditures Funded by the Government:

1950—22%
1965—21%
1980—39.2% (pp. 6–7)

The rise in health care expenditures has been dramatic; the rise in percentage of GNP for health care has been dramatic; and the rise in the role of public funding has been dramatic. The percentage of the gross domestic product (GDP, which is often used now in these measurements instead of GNP) for health care in the United States has continued to grow through the 1980s and into the 1990s (Levit et al. 1994):

1985—10.8%

1987—11.1%

1989—11.9%

1991—13.2%

1993—13.9%

The dollar figures and percentages represent more than curiosities for hospitals and physicians. A substantial reallocation of resources has taken place with the portion of the economy going to health care. There are good reasons for this.

—Inflation and population growth naturally make the dollar amounts, as opposed to percentages, larger.

—The advance in learning and the development of sophisticated technology make many more treatments available today and, consequently, more effective health care.

—The nature of the diseases people suffer has changed during this century: Much less infectious disease has given way to more acute illnesses. Chronic ailments may last decades and be treated for that long.

—People live longer.

—Increased availability of health care is provided by health insurance. Unlike several other industrialized countries, the United States has not had universal health insurance or care. The proportion of people covered increased substantially, however, with the coming of Medicare and Medicaid. Medicare and Medicaid have been great medical successes. They have permitted much greater access to care. The premiums for this medical insurance come via general taxation, and health care utilization was no longer linked to private payment. Socially, Medicare and Medicaid worked well. Financially, the systems created problems. When those eligible under these programs got sick or hurt, they would go to the doctor and/or go to the hospital. The physician and/or hospital ran the tests, did the laboratory work, took the x-rays, performed the surgery, applied radiotherapy, provided the meals, and nursed the patient. At the end of the process, the bills were totaled and sent to the government. The federal government, as well as the state government, then wrote a check to the doctor or to the hospital to reimburse the cost of the stay, diagnosis, treatment, and care. The method of payment based on cost reimbursement did not hinder the growth of total spending on health care.

As the 1970s came to an end, the country had been experiencing a high level of inflation and the federal government had had substantial budget deficits. As we have seen from the numbers, the federal government had become a prominent participant in health care, and a program was sought to lessen the growth of its economic role. How could that be addressed? What about the supply and demand for health care? What affects demand? We have already looked at factors like the aging population. Those factors certainly increase the demand for health care. What about price? Will less service be purchased at higher prices? That seems to be true for many things we buy. However, the demand for health services is seen to be rather inelastic. Elasticity has to do with the relative change in demand to a change in price. In our case of inelasticity, a rise in price would not decrease your purchasing by an equivalent percentage. For example, your doctor's fee goes up 25%. Your purchasing probably does not go down by as much as 25%. The demand is not absolutely inelastic. You could be expected to make some cuts in your demand. If you pay for your health insurance, for example, and the full health coverage includes physician services, hospitalization, drugs, dental care, eye examinations, corrective lenses, and so on, you might choose a less comprehensive level of coverage for a lower price. This can be seen with individuals and private insurance companies. Individuals choose to pay higher or lower premiums in anticipation of services offered.

What about the other side of the equation—supply? Hospitals and physicians are the primary suppliers of health care services in this country. In the 1980s the government chose to look at the suppliers of health care services and alter the method of reimbursement to them as a way to curtail the growing health care sector. Before this time hospitals and physicians were reimbursed by totaling the costs incurred for each patient. This made the hospital happy, this made the physician happy, and the patient was not disturbed. However, the budget deficit of the government was there. The solution devised was the prospective payment system. Treatment of a specific ailment, one might reason, should call for the use of certain resources. A determination is made of how much it should cost the health care providers, the hospital and physician, to treat a patient with a specific disease. Diagnostic related groups (DRGs) were the calculations of the average cost to treat different diseases, and that amount of money is what the government would send the provider for reimbursement. For example, a patient goes to the hospital for the surgical removal of a kidney stone. Let's say that he should be in the hospital four days, eat the meals, have his lab work, receive the anesthetic, have the operation, be nursed toward recovery, have his medical records updated, and be discharged. The government pays the providers $5,000. If the patient stays four days, the cost of the hospital and physician will be covered. If the patient stays three days, the providers may pocket the extra day's fee for themselves. If the patient stays five days, that extra day is coming out of the pockets of the hospital and physician. A hospital administrator may find that on balance, the hospital is losing money for the patients covered by these government programs. From the suppliers' point of view, they are shortchanged by the levels of reimbursement offered by the government. A more basic question now needed to be brought up. How do you know or determine what it costs to treat a patient for an illness? Perhaps there are some ailments that can fit into the prospective payment system without too much difficulty. However, the experience with DRGs did not always seem to be satisfactory.

MEDICAL EFFECTIVENESS AND HEALTH OUTCOMES

How can health care be made more effective or more efficient? How can people be treated and brought to better health with fewer resources expended? Preventive health care and education may be an answer. The reduction of certain behaviors such as smoking would lower morbidity in the population. One way to reduce the intensive use of the health care industry would be to initiate widespread health education and preventive medicine. Make it economically attractive for people to go for routine health checkups to catch problems before they progress and become more serious. Another initiative began that builds on the idea of the prospective payment system and DRGs. A new agency of the federal government has been created to address this issue. The Agency for Health Care Policy Research (AHCPR) aims to study health treatments and health outcomes (Clevesy and Smith 1993). Look back in Chapter 4 to the discussion about the NLM collection development policy. There, one of the examples given for an area of the collection was "Health Services Research," defined as "the scientific study of the effect of health care delivery and management on health care access, quality, and cost." The AHCPR would like to quantify the access people have to health care, the effectiveness of the health care they receive, and the cost of that health care. The systematic study of the effectiveness of health care is a new and challenging role for a government agency. When you go to the doctor, the treatments you are given are pretty much determined by what your doctor knows and what his or her experiences have been. There is no guarantee that your doctor knows and uses state-of-the-art diagnostic methods or treatments for your particular illness. This discussion takes us right back to us, the health sciences librarians. Are doctors getting the information they need? When new procedures and techniques are developed so rapidly, how do practitioners really know what works? Such questions explain why this agency as well as others is developing "practice parameters" or "clinical practice guidelines." The guidelines give the clinicians the state-of-the-art information they are expected to know and use. Skeptics call this "cookbook medicine." Proponents see it as a way to implement methods that have proven useful.

How have these methods proven themselves useful? Studies involving "outcomes research" are the plans for the 1990s. Take coronary bypass surgery as an example. This technique was developed and surgeons started using the procedure in large numbers. Patients found relief from the pain and many physicians believed the procedure would increase patient survival. Not until large-scale systematic studies were conducted years later was it found that life expectancy was no different for bypass patients than for those who had medical management (Coronary Artery Surgery Study Group 1983). Most procedures doctors perform have not undergone rigorous large-scale testing. The incentive to do outcomes research and develop practice parameters is derived from the desire to provide better medical care and to do that in more efficient and less wasteful ways. The all-important question is this: Does the information from the literature apply to the specific patient? Should the doctor use the clinical practice guideline for the patient he or she is treating? Take a look at the series from *JAMA* ''Users' Guides to the Medical Literature. VIII. How to Use Clinical Practice Guidelines'' (Wilson et al. 1995). To find more information on health services research, use the Health Services/Technology Assessment Research (HSTAR) database from NLM. Citations are taken from MEDLINE, Health Planning and Administration, and CATLINE. Other articles, technical reports, and government documents are included, too. The National Library of Medicine also intends to include newspaper articles and abstracts from meetings.

THE HOSPITAL'S ECONOMIC HEALTH AND YOU

The changes in the 1980s made quick and extensive impacts on our institutions. Hospital admissions went down, 10.3% from 1983 to 1986, and average length of stay in the hospital decreased by 17% in those years (Guterman et al. 1988, 69). Hospitals have closed. The 1993–94 edition of *Hospital Statistics* (American Hospital Association 1993) gives the number of community hospitals in 1982 (5,801) and the number for 1992 (5,292) (p. xxxvii). The closures over the ten years have not been uniformly distributed. The number of urban hospitals decreased by 1.1%, whereas the number for rural hospitals went down 17.2% (p. xxxviii). The difficulties extend far beyond the hospitals that have closed. Many hospitals that have survived continue on tight budgets and recurring deficits. There have been many hospital mergers that were motivated largely to improve the hospital's financial situations. The economics of running a hospital have made for difficult decisions, and the impact on many hospital libraries has been negative. One immediate economic issue for the library is that it is not a direct revenue producing service. Take, for example, a nonlibrary service in the hospital. A patient is given respiratory therapy. The charges for the use of the supplies and equipment and the pay for the respiratory therapist are part of a patient's bill. The cost is direct and quantifiable. What about you? You supply information to health care providers that enable them to do their jobs better and more efficiently. You know this. They may have a vague notion of it. However, how do you quantify the cost of your services and parcel out to each patient's care (and bill) the mental acquisition that the health care provider received and used? This is a real problem for the librarian in an era of very close cost analysis.

Until several years ago hospitals that treated Medicaid and Medicare patients were under a regulation that stipulated the presence of a library. The Health Care Financing Administration (HCFA) revised those regulations and eliminated the requirement (Davies 1982). The Joint Commission on Accreditation of Healthcare Organizations (JCAHO) is the main accrediting body of hospitals, and it does include requirements for the provision of library services. In the past, the requirements that related to the library were not considered high priority. In other words, hospitals did not get into much trouble for failing to supply adequate library service. The commisson has revised its standards, and library service can now be a real factor in the information management standard. This is encouraging. Nonetheless, the hard facts remain. However much we might like regulatory agencies or legislative bodies to recognize us and require our services, we are still going to have to show our contribution to our clientele and, in particular, our administrators.

You need a little history of the hospital to understand your environment. Here is a very little history. The hospital was not nearly so prominent a participant in health care a century ago. In the nineteenth century the one place you did not want to be when you were sick was the hospital. That was the place for the poor who had nowhere else to go. All but the poor were treated at home. Nurses were often given the charge of running the hospital. Around the start of the twentieth century, advances in surgery and infection control made hospitals a safer place to be. The middle class came for care, and the physicians took over the hospitals. Professional managers joined the physicians in joint authority for the management of hospitals, and hospitals became more important in medical education, too. Through the years hospitals became less central to the education of nurses. More and more nurses earned their degrees outside the hospital: two-year associate's degrees at community colleges and four-year baccalaureate degrees at colleges and universities. For our part, before the Medical Library Assistance Act (discussed later in the chapter), many hospital libraries did not have much to offer in terms of resources or trained staff or links to information outside the four walls.

In 1946 the Hospital Survey and Construction Act, usually referred to as the Hill-Burton Act, provided for funding of community hospitals. The intent was to provide sufficient hospital facilities throughout the country, with the needs of rural areas foremost in mind. Funding from the government for education, research, and facilities became such an integral part over time that efforts at reform in years of retrenchment have meant momentous impacts on all involved. Starting in the 1960s Medicaid and Medicare spending meant that hospitals often did not have to treat the indigent for free. They were reimbursed with real monies. With the shortage of physicians, the federal government started paying medical schools money for the education of medical students. This was a great help to the budgets of the medical schools. The reimbursement to hospitals for Medicaid and Medicare patients helped pay for graduate medical education in the form of residencies of physicians in the hospitals. Money for research from the NIH came showering down on faculty at medical schools across the country. The universities enjoyed this in that their prestige was heightened by the research of their employees. In direct financial terms, the research grants from NIH paid the salary of those faculty. Not having to spend university money to pay the medical faculty, universities had those resources available for other purposes (i.e., budget relief). All these outcomes and more made numerous impacts on the relationships of the parties involved and on the flow of funds. Therefore when the flow of money for medical students was halted by the federal government and when the DRG method of reimbursement for Medicaid and Medicare was put in place, available monies to spread around dried up. The hospitals were deprived of a lot of their funds. Medical education, which also depended on funds indirectly from Medicare and Medicaid, found difficulties, too. The relationships between the practice of medicine in the hospitals and the teaching of medicine by the medical schools was much easier when the parties had enough money. When resources became tight, the real differences in the roles of the hospital and medical school could be seen in their disputes over who would get the money. The trend away from inpatient hospitalization and toward ambulatory care brings with it more changes in roles of institutions and flows of monies. It even calls into question the very existence of the hospital as the central health care facility. In addition, all those factors in increasing the size of the health care sector—the aging population is one prominent feature—are not going away. Does this information really need to be in a book on health sciences librarianship? It is here because the economic environment is so important to us. The hospital will continue to be pressured this way and that. You, as the hospital librarian, will feel the effects of this dynamic situation.

The doctor is caught in the middle of the pressures to keep costs lower, provide good health care that involves use of resources, and worrying about skimping on utilization for fear of malpractice actions. These issues have a way of coming up in the everyday practice of medicine. From a professor of medical ethics:

> The utilization review committee of a major teaching hospital found that one cardiologist's patients suffering acute myocardial infarctions consistently had hospitalization expenses far exceeding those of his colleagues' patients. While the average stay for such patients at the hospital was 13.1 days, this physician's patients stayed on average 18.2 days. The average cost of hospitalization at this institution for acute myocardial infarction was $10,257, while this physician's patients averaged costs of $14,132. The physician in question was thus an *outlier*—one whose patients consistently showed substantial deviation from mean resource consumption. (Veatch 1986, 32)

Will outcomes studies and practice parameters help in these situations, or will the individual problems of each patient undermine a drive to more systematic medical practices? Being a doctor involves more than the art and science of medicine and biology. Doses of economics, politics, and administrative regulations are also prescribed.

MEDICAL LIBRARY ASSISTANCE ACT AND THE REGIONAL MEDICAL LIBRARY PROGRAM

Running your library today means that you need to understand the programs and resources available to health sciences libraries. You should know how the networks and programs came to be and how they have evolved. In Chapter 2 we saw that NLM had great success with MEDLARS. The National Library of Medicine had achieved an important goal in producing timely access to the medical literature, and the medical literature contained breakthroughs (e.g., open heart surgery, vaccine for polio). A continuing doubt, though, acted as a drag on the feelings of progress in the medical community. What good were all the scientific and medical advances if they were not known about in the community? if the local physicians were not using the new knowledge? What could be done to inform the health care practitioners? In addition, a shortage of physicians was perceived in the country. New medical schools were being built. Was there proper support for the medical faculty, researchers, and students as well as the practicing physicians? The answer was no. Libraries were inadequate and not up to the task of delivering the wealth of new information. They often did not have up-to-date collections, the staff was not well-trained enough in the medical literature, and the funding was insufficient. Senator Lister Hill declared:

> While justifiably proud of this magnificent institution here in Bethesda, we cannot ignore overwhelming evidence to the effect that medical libraries in other parts of the country have neither the financing, the equipment, nor the personnel to disseminate quickly to the practitioner of medicine the life-saving bounty of newly acquired research knowledge. We are not talking now of books and journals for future reference—we are talking of medical findings whose worth is meaningless unless they are applied to the disease problems of our time. (Hill 1966, 82)

The Medical Library Assistance Act (MLAA), Public Law 89–291, became law in 1965 (Cummings and Corning 1971). Its goal was to improve facilities and services across the nation. It empowered NLM to make grants to organizations outside the library. The act authorized the establishment of a Regional Medical Library Program (RMLP), and considerable debate ensued on how to organize this program. Existing strong medical libraries around the country were selected to be regional medical libraries. Funds, training, services, and support flowed from NLM to the regional medical libraries and through them to medical libraries throughout the country. Eleven areas were set up and continued until the early 1980s, when it was reorganized into seven regions. In 1991 one of the consolidations that had been made in 1982 was split off into two. Currently there are eight regions:

1. Middle Atlantic (Delaware, New Jersey, New York, Pennsylvania)
2. Southeast-Atlantic (Alabama, Florida, Georgia, Maryland, Mississippi, North Carolina, South Carolina, Tennessee, Virginia, West Virginia, District of Columbia, Puerto Rico, Virgin Islands)
3. Greater Midwest (Illinois, Indiana, Iowa, Kentucky, Michigan, Minnesota, North Dakota, Ohio, South Dakota, Wisconsin)
4. Midcontinental (Colorado, Kansas, Missouri, Nebraska, Utah, Wyoming)

5. South Central (Arkansas, Louisiana, New Mexico, Oklahoma, Texas)
6. Pacific Northwest (Alaska, Idaho, Montana, Oregon, Washington)
7. Pacific Southwest (Arizona, California, Hawaii, Nevada, U.S. Pacific Territories)
8. New England (Connecticut, Maine, Massachusetts, New Hampshire, Rhode Island, Vermont)

Funds were made available to help build collections. The training of medical librarians was facilitated by paying educational expenses for librarians and library school students. Search analysts located in the regions were trained by NLM. Via the RMLP, NLM also tremendously facilitated the process of interlibrary loan. Prior to this time, interlibrary loan had been an ongoing activity in all types of libraries. However, it was often a slow process and not a satisfactory service for the medical community. The timely transfer of information was the prime goal of the Medical Library Assistance Act. How might the interlibrary loan process be improved? Make it free—free to the participants, anyway. Of course, libraries would incur expenses in staff time and supplies in filling the interlibrary loan requests, but NLM would cover the costs. Local libraries, such as hospital libraries, would send their requests, which were usually for journal articles, to the resource library. The resource library was often the closest medical school library. If the resource library did not own the publication, it would send the request on to the regional medical library. Then NLM would fully reimbursed the regional medical library or the resource library for the cost of supplying the loan, and reimbursement was also available to the library that made referrals.

This program was extremely popular, and a great volume of article photocopies crossed the country in the mails. It was a great success. The literature flowed freely. It was so successful that one medical publisher, Williams & Wilkins, brought suit against NLM for copyright violation. The publisher contended that the amount of the photocopying done at NLM, which received referrals from the regional medical libraries, was so high that it was replacing the subscriptions the libraries would otherwise have had with the publisher. Williams & Wilkins did not win the case, but the decisions from the courts came with very narrow margins. This episode and case were factors considered in the debate that resulted in the 1976 Copyright Law. Over the next several years NLM gradually pulled back its financial support for interlibrary loans. Libraries took over the cost of the transactions, and by this time the system was firmly in place. The RMLP served the local libraries in other ways. It supported training for online searching, and the regional medical libraries helped with reference service backup. It supplied consulting services and classes on managing hospital libraries. The program also offered support and expertise in helping states and regions develop local union lists of journal holdings. This was very important in facilitating local interlibrary loan transactions (Bunting 1987).

NLM THROUGH THE 1980s AND 1990s

The next step in facilitating interlibrary loan was taken with the introduction of DOCLINE. Libraries throughout the country reported their journal holdings to NLM through their regional libraries. The database of these holdings is SERHOLD. Libraries log into DOCLINE in much the same way they have been accessing MEDLINE. Before using the system, each library will have entered a list of libraries to which it would normally wish to send its requests. In this system, the requesting library does not need to check union lists or other finding aids for each request to determine which library to go to. DOCLINE automatically and randomly selects a library that has that journal and sends your request. Another method to facilitate the flow of information has been the training of health professionals in the use of online systems. Grateful Med is the software developed specifically for the use of end users in searching the MEDLARS databases. It helps the users identify the journal articles they need. Loansome Doc is a program added to the Grateful Med software that gives health professionals a way to order the full journal articles from a library directly from their literature search. The next steps are on the horizon—direct electronic access to the full text of the documents.

Other programs at NLM include the Lister Hill National Center of Biomedical Communications and the National Center for Biotechnology Information. The products and services initiated by NLM have played important roles in our libraries. The DeBakey Report in the 1960s (United States. President's Commission on Heart Disease, Cancer and Stroke 1964–65) provided the impetus for the Medical Library Assistance Act and the Regional Medical Library Program. In the late 1980s Michael DeBakey chaired a panel to look at this issue again and to "find techniques for disseminating to health professionals the information they need to minister to their patients in the most efficient and effective way possible" (National Library of Medicine. Board of Regents 1989, 2). These steps are bringing us closer to the goal, namely, to quickly and conveniently getting information to people who need it. The newly renamed Regional Medical Library Program—now National Network of Libraries of Medicine or NN/LM—continues to serve us. However, for a number of years, additional organizations and online and CD-ROM vendors beyond this library network have begun to take an increasing role in our computer searching of the literature. Now we are also using other means of acquiring individual journal articles with document delivery supplementing interlibrary loan. For up-to-date information on NLM programs, check its fact sheets available on its home page or Gopher.

MEDICAL EDUCATION, BIOMEDICAL RESEARCH, AND OUR LITERATURE

Medical education and research provide much of the demand for our services. Research generates new information for our supply of literature. In looking at the history of medical librarianship, a very brief note about the history of medical education is needed to show the evolution of this demand and supply. The state of medical education in 1900 was very different from the situation today. At that time, there were many proprietary medical schools. Often the instruction consisted of a series of lectures without any opportunity for laboratory work. The teachers were mainly practicing physicians who taught in their spare time. Admission requirements to attend many of these schools were minimal. Therefore, large numbers of physicians were inadequately prepared for their occupation. At the same time, there were several medical schools affiliated with universities that had stringent requirements and adequate facilities. It was not difficult to see that parts of medical education could be reformed. Abraham Flexner was commissioned by the Carnegie Foundation for the Advancement of Teaching to investigate the state of medical education in the United States. He traveled throughout the country visiting medical schools. The Flexner Report (1910) was the turning point for medical education. His recommendations were accepted and acted upon: Students applying to medical school were required to have a baccalaureate degree; science and laboratory courses were required as part of medical instruction; medical schools needed to have full-time teachers—people dedicated to education and not just teaching as a spare-time endeavor. Criticism of medical education has been continuous to this day. However, after the Flexner Report, changes were made. Very quickly, many of the proprietary schools either closed or merged with an institution of higher learning. Medical education improved. The stipulation of maintaining a full-time faculty had other consequences, especially for us in the library. Opportunities for research were now available. Full-time faculty members in a university setting are expected to do research. This further advanced the state of knowledge of medicine and was a great impetus to increasing the volume of information. Doing research meant writing about your research. The publish-or-perish commentary held true for the medical school as well as the rest of the university. This provided the opportunity to write more, and the growth of the medical literature accelerated. The result of all this is that physicians and medical students now have a lot more to learn.

The current era begins with World War II. At that time, the federal government started to provide tremendous sums of money to support basic and applied research in the sciences (e.g., the Manhattan Project). Research had certainly been conducted before World War II at universities and laboratories throughout the country. The research there had been along traditional lines, with the goal of enlarging the information in an area of learning. Federal government spending had not been a large factor. "To summarize, the scientific and technological requirements of World War II resulted not only in an unprecedented level of governmental expenditure, but also in the rise of targeted, interdisciplinary research and development—mission-oriented research" (Adams 1981, 19).

> The single most telling piece of evidence about the changing scale of biomedical research is revealed in the total expenditures for the two years 1940 and 1987. In 1940 total outlays for biomedical research amounted to $45 million. The 1987 figure is estimated at $16.2 billion, 360 times the earlier figure. In constant (inflation-adjusted) dollars, the increase is close to fortyfold. (Ginzberg and Dutka 1989, 1)

Biomedical research is an expensive endeavor. The federal government has taken over the prominent role of funding. In earlier years, philanthropy had provided a significant percentage. Its portion of the whole has gone down. Industry, notably the pharmaceutical companies and their research into drugs, has an important role in biomedical research, too.

The top source of government-sponsored funding for biomedicine is the NIH. At NIH, the proposals from scientists are evaluated by a process of peer review. Each proposal is examined by experts in that specific area of research. The experts will make a judgment on the merit of the research proposal. Among the factors the reviewers consider are these: (1) Is the hypothesis well thought out and will it likely yield significant new information? (2) Is the experiment well designed with adequate controls and suitable methods? (3) Is the investigator adequately prepared for this research with a background of training and a familiarity with the literature? (4) Are the resources and facilities adequate to conduct the research? Applications are assigned an overall rating (Strickland 1989). Let us say that a proposal received a very high rating. Whether the project is funded then becomes a question of how much money is available and how many other requests received an even higher approval score. During the 1950s and early 1960s, federal biomedical research increased at a rate of 18% annually. That has not been the situation for many years. The process is very competitive, and many very highly evaluated proposals are not funded (Marshall 1994).

With the competition for funding, controversies arise. How much money should be put into large projects? Will the extensive funding of a big science endeavor take resources away from other worthy projects? These are questions of policy that are not necessarily decided on the basis of science. Just as war is too important to leave to the generals, the health of individuals in our society is too important to leave to the health professionals. The funding for the war on cancer in the 1970s was not unanimously hailed by the research community. The big science projects of the 1990s are the research on AIDS and the Human Genome Project. Again, unanimity is not present in the biomedical research community. Disagreements arise over the basic question of economics: the division of the relatively scarce resources and the diversion away from other deserving projects. Not only may the allocations for research projects be contested but the funding for its indirect costs may bring about controversy. The overhead costs of doing research include administration (e.g., paying the bills), physical plant (e.g., heating the buildings), and libraries (e.g., information services). Parenthetically, it would be useful to determine if appropriate overhead funds arrived in the library. That could be a source of controversy for us. The more publicized controversy has been the variable rates of overhead charged by different universities and the disparate types of items charged to overhead (Rosenzweig 1991).

Another controversy relating to funding is misconduct by health care professionals (Woolf 1987). Were physicians to any real extent taking advantage of Medicaid in the 1970s to claim reimbursement for more than they were entitled? What about biomedical research? With the competition for funding so strong, have there been more than the handful of reported cases of "doctored" data in research studies? One of the more widely publicized cases of fraud was that of John Darsee at Harvard University. He was regarded as brilliant and incredibly productive. He published close to 100 papers and abstracts in two years (Broad and Wade 1982). It turned out that Darsee was fabricating his data. He had his papers published widely, and others were then using his findings in their work. Although the extent of this type of thing is unknown, this, too, is a part of the background environment that you should understand.

With the funding secured, the work can move along. Biomedical research is done in a variety of settings. Physicians in hospitals are involved in clinical protocols with their patients. Universities, private companies, and not-for-profit companies are settings for many test tube (in vitro) and animal (in vivo) studies. In addition, epidemiological projects are undertaken with surveys and manipulations of gathered data.

OUTCOMES RESEARCH FOR THE LIBRARY

This brings us back to you again. Your role is to help physicians, other health professionals, and students in their acquisition of knowledge over their entire careers. The health care system does have problems. Many people feel that too much is spent on health care and we are not getting enough for our dollar. The system seems inefficient and wasteful. Solutions to one problem seem to worsen others. However, there are often solutions out there that people do not avail themselves of. A physician cannot now begin by ordering every laboratory test and diagnostic procedure under the sun. He or she has to find the one(s) that will most likely yield the desired data. This type of information that can guide the health care providers in their decisions is what we often have in the library and could provide to the practitioner. "When the hospital's library service is good enough so that its information influences decision-making throughout the hospital, then the value of this information will show in terms of improved patient care, better use of resources and overall lowered costs" (Jensen 1981, 45). Our assistance is not limited to the hospital. There is plenty to do in the medical school, too. There are an array of problems that academic medicine has never really addressed: "skyrocketing expenditures for medical care, substandard indexes of population health, uneven quality of care, an unfavorable geographic and specialty mix of physicians, and widespread disability from long-term medical and psychiatric problems'' (Schroeder, Zones, and Showstack 1989, 803). The academic health centers have done great things in the roles that they have chosen. They are the centers for the impressive biomedical research in this country. They could be encouraged to extend their research capabilities to confront these difficult medical and societal problems.

Although we have not thought carefully in these terms before, we need to determine more specifically how our service to our patrons makes a difference in their work. Anecdotal evidence may help. However, our own kind of outcomes research would be better. The National Library of Medicine is developing the Critical Incident Technique that may help us. It is ''a systematic approach for obtaining and analyzing substantial numbers of detailed reports of behaviors leading to successful or unsuccessful outcomes on a task or process'' (Lindberg et al. 1993, 3124). This is an organized attempt to go beyond the anecdotal evidence of testimonials of doctors coming back to us to tell us how useful our information was to the treating of a patient.

The time has passed when we can judge the quality of our library and its service by the number of books and journal subscriptions and by the size of our budget. We need to see and show how what we do makes a difference. King (1987) oversaw an eight-hospital study in Chicago, and Marshall (1992) conducted a fifteen-hospital program in Rochester, New York, to determine the impact library services have on how doctors treat their patients. In Rochester, physicians included in a large sample were asked to request information from their hospital libraries. The questions were to pertain to patient cases on which they were then working. After receiving the information, they were asked to evaluate the impact that information had on what they decided to do in the care of the patients. Among the findings were the impact on the advice given to the patient (71.6% changed) and the choice of diagnostic test (50.5% changed). This multicenter study (to put it in the words of a MeSH publication type) presents the findings that we like to hear, but we need to go further. ''Another limitation of both the Chicago and Rochester studies is that the results are based on self-reporting. While physicians, as key decision makers in the health care system, are in the best position to evaluate the impact of library information on their own clinical decisions, it would be desirable to have confirming data from other sources'' (Marshall 1992, 177). In the current era, the best-case scenario shows library service contributing both to better patient outcomes and to cost savings (Klein et al. 1994).

TOTAL QUALITY MANAGEMENT, JCAHO, AND LIBRARY STANDARDS

In a sense, hospital libraries have been indebted to the JCAHO for including the library in its *Accreditation Manual for Hospitals*. Beyond inclusion, librarians are looking forward to more rigorous requirements for the library from JCAHO. The commission has incorporated portions of MLA's own *Standards for Hospital Libraries* (Medical Library Association 1994). In addition, the hospital library is moving into the system of quality service recommended by JCAHO. A few years ago the plan that hospitals embraced was quality assurance (QA). Now there is a another idea. The following comes from the American Hospital Association journal, *Hospitals and Health Networks*:

> Pressured by local, state and national health care reform initiatives, hospitals are searching for ways to provide more cost-effective care. This is seen in a variety of patient care restructuring, clinical re-engineering and value improvement programs. But by far the most comprehensive and enthusiastic response to efforts to improve quality while containing or lowering costs is reflected in hospitals' commitment to continuous quality improvement/total quality management (CQI/TQM). (The Quality March 1993, 52)

The standards developed by the MLA (1994) for hospital libraries have integrated the ideas of CQI/TQM into the library's mission and activities. In general, TQM works like this: In order to supply better service, you need to know what functions your clientele perform and the information needs they have. It is up to you to find that out. Then you need to determine the best way to serve those needs. This is not a goal to be achieved and set aside. Achieving it is a continuous process because you will need to evaluate the changing needs of your clientele and the changing state of the art of information services.

Specifically, how can TQM be applied? Through surveys and interviews you have discovered, for example, that your patrons need health care business information. ''This clientele is unlikely to be satisfied with long lists of bibliographic references. Nor will they want to hear tales of drastic reductions in journal subscriptions due to the last five years of budget cuts. Many medical library collections are largely unprepared to meet demands for business management sources'' (Snow 1993, 103). You evaluate what you have been doing in this area of business information—little. With the TQM model, ''benchmarking'' is your search for how others perform this task the best. If their solutions fit your circumstance, copy it. It should be emphasized that libraries have traditionally focused on documents. That is, we have found the publications that we believe will meet the meets of our patrons. In many instances, what the patron really wants is information that answers their questions—that is, they want the data, not the literature that contains the data. This may be the case with our traditional clientele of physicians and researchers and nurses as well as the administrators. Fortunately for us this happens to be the time that the data are ''out there'' and increasingly available through our node on the electronic network. We need to become familiar with, understand, and use the databases, telecommunications, and computerized networks of biomedicine. To meet their needs, we need to know more about our users. We need to investigate, in particular, those users beyond the doctors and researchers who have been the main audience so far. ''At the turn of the twentieth century physicians accounted for about one out of every three health workers. At the beginnings of the 1980s the comparable ratio is approximately one out of sixteen'' (Ginzberg 1983, 479). Many of these positions are recent additions to the health care field and came into being with new services developed from technological innovations. Other occupations have been around a long time but have had changing roles in the delivery of health care.

WHAT ABOUT NURSES AND ALLIED HEALTH?

Although medical doctors have been the central focus of our activities over the years, they do not represent the largest group in health care work. Nurses are number one. There are over 2 million nurses. Nursing has been a predominantly female occupation throughout its history. In the nineteenth century, nursing was an added responsibility for women. Wives, mothers, daughters, aunts, and so on, took care of the ailing members of the family. People were cared for at home. When help was needed to care for the patient, a ''professed'' nurse was hired. Formal education was not the usual road to nursing. She ''professed'' that she was a nurse. Eventually, programs were set up to train nurses, and hospitals set up these programs. The nursing students employed by the hospitals spent most of their time working in the hospitals and very little in a classroom. Most of the staff of the hospital was composed of student nurses. When a nurse finished her program, she was expected to find employment as a nurse outside of the hospital.

Debates have continued on many aspects of nursing, with education a central issue. Who should do the educating of nurses? What about other levels of nurses (e.g., licensed practical nurses) (Reverby 1987)? Medical librarians have a certification process set up through their professional association, the MLA. It is a factor that libraries may choose to use when hiring medical librarians. However, certification for librarians is voluntary. You do not need to be certified to be a medical librarian. An employer may or may not require it. In contrast to that situation, most health care workers must be licensed by a governmental body to practice their profession. Today, after a nurse earns her (or sometimes his) degree (diploma or associate or baccalaureate), she takes a test, NCLEX-RN to enable her to practice nursing in the state (Matassarin-Jacobs 1989). All fifty states require this.

Another area of concern is the periodic shortages of nurses. Many explanations are given for this. There is a greater demand for nurses because the patients who do go to the hospital now are sicker than before. Many patients who in earlier decades would have been put in the hospital are now treated as outpatients. There is a fairly large turnover in certain types of nursing, such as acute care. Nursing homes naturally present another demand for nurses. The compensation for nurses may be a factor, too. Nurses may start at a high salary, but the potential for greater income over the years is small unless they leave the bedside and go into supervision and administration. The pay for veteran nurses is not much greater than for new nurses, and this leads to some disenchantment.

Unlike times not long ago, nursing is just one of countless occupations a woman may choose. Also, nursing is still mostly a female occupation. "Ninety-seven percent of nurses are female and 91% are non-Hispanic whites" (Friedman 1990, 2851). What will happen in the future? Will the nurse take on more of the duties traditionally performed by the physician? The ongoing advance of technology makes the nurse continue to grow in the job in order to use the advanced equipment. Will the parts of the job not having to do with the care of the patient—running errands, doing the paperwork, sending orders—still take up much of the nurse's time? During the current era some perceive an oversupply of physicians. What will that mean for the nursing role? In an earlier time, a physician shortage, gave nurses an opportunity to fill part of that void. Will physicians be less likely to yield some of their traditional functions to nurses now that there is no void?

The cooperative work of nurses with physicians has been important to health care for a long time. What should the relationship be between nurses and physicians? And what is the division of labor between physicians and nurses? How about the role of nurse practitioners and physician assistants? What is the role of nurses? This has continued to change. The relationship has been characterized this way:

> Nurses were to be bold, have initiative, and be responsible for making important recommendations, while at the same time they had to seem passive. In short, nurses were to make recommendations, but their recommendations had to appear to be initiated by the physician. The cardinal rule of the game was that open disagreement between the players had to be avoided at all costs. (Stein, Watts, and Howell 1990, 546)

Today nurses are less likely to go along with this game. Another thing that nurses are less likely to do, it seems, is use the library. In a study of their hospital, Bunyan and Lutz (1991) found that nurses made up only 6% of their users. That contrasts with the fact that nurses were 31% of the hospital's employees.

Other employees who have underutilized the library are those found under the umbrella term "allied health." The status and variety of duties continue to evolve here, too, and we need to know more about the needs of these employees. For example, which group would you say has a professional association with the name American Health Information Management Association (AHIMA)? What might this be? The group of hospital library directors? Perhaps the directors of the medical school libraries? No, that group is the Association of Academic Health Sciences Library Directors (AAHSLD). The AHIMA was formerly AMRA, the American Medical Records Association. This seems a bit confusing. In years past when you introduced yourself as a medical librarian, more than a few people would think you were a medical records librarian. In the interim, the people in medical records changed their title to medical records administrator. Now we see a further change to health information managers. What do we as health sciences librarians think of this? We have always assumed that we have the central role in health information and that we have the knowledge and skills for that title.

There will be demand for health care information for the foreseeable future. The health care occupations are working in a growth industry. The Bureau of Labor Statistics projects the following growth (Gradler and Schrammel 1994):

	1992 estimated employment	**Growth in numbers 1992–2005**	**Growth in percentage 1992–2005**
Registered Nurses	1,835,000	765,000	42
Physicians	556,000	195,000	35
Pharmacists	163,000	47,000	29
Physical Therapists	90,000	79,000	88
Physicians Assistants	58,000	20,000	34

How many health sciences librarians are there? From NLM's *The Education and Training of Health Sciences Librarians* comes this assessment (National Library of Medicine 1995d, 5):

7,000–10,000 health sciences librarians in over 3,600 health-related organizations in the U.S. and Canada

46% work in hospital libraries

25% work in academic health sciences centers

Bachelor's degree: 21%, English or journalism; 19%, social sciences; 15%, biomedical or biological sciences; 14%, education

Here is the gist of it:

Health Care—a growth industry

Health Care Information—a growth industry

Health Sciences Librarians—?

What is the employment outlook for the health sciences librarian? The answer depends on how we adapt to serve the needs of our users and how much we expand our user population beyond the doctors, nurses, researchers, and students.

THE INFORMATION NEEDS OF THE HOSPITAL ADMINISTRATOR

You, as the hospital librarian, are an employee of the hospital. Most of the people who work in the hospital are employees of the hospital. However, most of the physicians working in the hospital are not employees of the hospital. They request hospital privileges in order to treat their patients there. The physicians are linked to a hospital through contractual arrangements. Doctors have been, continue to be, and, even with the changes in health care will be the key health care providers. Although the physicians are not employees of the hospital, they largely determine how the hospital's resources are used because they direct the treatment of the patient. The hospital needs doctors. Also, doctors need hospitals, a place with the expensive equipment and support for patient care. The health care issues debated by the country also reflect the conflict between the medical staff and the hospital. The diminished rate of reimbursement from government programs and the inability to obtain the latest equipment for a hospital conflict with the physician's goal of treating the patient as extensively as needed with the most useful tools (Shortell 1991). Administrators endeavor to keep costs down; physicians need to use resources. True, the ultimate focus of all parties is on the health of the patient and good patient care. However, many economic, political, and personality issues need to be resolved in order to achieve that end.

Another audience we need to serve, but often have not, is comprised of the administrators. These are the people who run the hospital in all its aspects except clinical care. They oversee the fiscal situation of the hospital, the departments, and the employees. The hospital administrator has a continuous need for information. Administrators will be much more understanding of your role if they can get some of the benefits of your service. You can make ''economic'' contributions in many ways. For example, legislative actions relating to health care are important. The administrator must keep up on the regulations issued by agencies of governments. We may employ many of the tools at our disposal in this effort. One current awareness service offered by hospital librarians entails scanning current issues of journals for articles they know would be of interest to individual physicians. The same may be done for administrators. Information may be culled from the receipt of newspapers, periodicals, and other sources. A news publication made up of the sources you scan can be sent to interested parties each day. You do not need to limit yourself to prestigious publications covered in the journal literature of Chapter 1. For example, regulations issued by the federal government have ongoing and important impacts on the running of the hospital. You may have a subscription to the *Federal Register*, or you could look at it on the Internet. Each business day the *Federal Register* has a few hundred pages of regulations and announcements of proposed regulations. The hospital administration needs to know these things not only in order to obey the rules but also to lobby the agencies for changes they do and do not want to take place. You have an important opportunity here. Don't limit your sources to the printed items in your library. The hundreds of electronic databases and services to which you have access have a world of news information, business advice, and political insights.

Here is one scenario. Your boss, Mr. Lindsay, is the vice-president in charge of research and information services of the hospital. He is concerned about a recent piece of legislation and the follow-up regulations. The Animal Welfare Act and amendments address the issue of animals in biomedical research. This is also an issue that has been covered in the popular press. Researchers are confident that they have been using animals in a proper manner. Mr. Lindsay needs to know, however, the emerging regulations for the hospital's laboratory animals. There is a committee in the hospital, the Animal Care Committee, that is set up for this purpose, and the committee also needs information. Interestingly, among the directives you find is a recommendation from the U.S. Department of Agriculture (USDA). The USDA suggests that literature searches be done (1) to make sure that the research involving animals is not a duplication of research already done and (2) to learn techniques in animal experimentation to lessen pain and suffering. The USDA specifies that a search of MEDLINE will address the former and a search of AGRICOLA (USDA's database) will address the latter. This is not really surprising. Before researchers embark on a project, they need to research the literature to make sure their experiment has not already been done. They are not likely to get funded if it has. The USDA's recommendation serves to formalize the process. The USDA's second object is new, though: to search the literature for less invasive or painful techniques. Admittedly, for us in the library this is a rather self-serving example. However, it does show clearly a role for us to play. Our service to the administrators can be the same as it has been to the clinicians, students, and researchers. Along with money, information is what the hospital administrator needs most. Hospital administrators do know this. They are concerned about their information systems. When they think of "information systems," they more likely see their computerized payroll or patient billing processes. Too infrequently do they think of the library as an information provider for them. You can demonstrate your usefulness for them. You must take this as part of your mission.

THE LARGER ENVIRONMENT: HEALTH CARE ASSOCIATIONS AND ORGANIZATIONS

The environment in which we do our jobs extends beyond our libraries, hospitals, and schools. The health sciences librarian needs to be familiar with numerous associations and organizations. Their activities and policies have an impact on the delivery of health care and research. These organizations are at all levels: local, state, national, and international. Private and governmental organizations play roles. Look at the seventh edition of the *Medical and Health Information Directory* (Boyden 1994). Volume 1 in the three-volume set has 1659 pages. Pages 1–476 include descriptions of 4,235 national and international associations. Here is a sampling of the entries:

American Board of Medical Specialties—oversees the separate specialty boards that establish standards for education and qualifications of physicians

American College of Physicians—for physicians in internal medicine (70,000 members)

American Dental Association—professional society of dentists (140,000 members)

American Geriatrics Society—for physicians specializing in problems of aging (6,022 members)

American Hospital Association—interests include hospital administration and health care delivery (54,500 members)

American Medical Association—the large national association of physicians (271,000 members)

American Nurses' Association—association of registered nurses (200,000 members)

American Optometric Association (29,000 members)

American Psychological Association (70,000 members)

American Public Health Association (31,500 members)

This sample is but a token listing of a few national organizations and societies that have roles in health care. There are thousands more of these and thousands more of state and local organizations, too. In addition, governmental organizations exist at the local, state, and federal levels. They perform many functions. The organizations (e.g., American Lung Association) may be sources of information for you and your patrons. They provide standards and regulations (e.g., Joint Commission on Accreditation of Healthcare Organizations). Some, like the National Head Injury Foundation, are for the support of patients. Some are for licensure, like the Kentucky State Board of Medical Licensure. States also have departments to collect vital data (e.g., Minnesota Department of Public Health State Registrar and Center for Health Statistics). Agencies such as the Health Care Financing Administration also oversee large federal programs. Agencies like NIH direct the biomedical research efforts funded by the federal government. The National Institutes of Health itself includes the National Institute of Aging, the National Institute of Dental Research, the National Eye Institute, and the National Cancer Institute, among other subagencies. These organizations will have a large impact on what you do and on the work of the patrons you are serving. You will become familiar with many of them.

MEDICAL LIBRARY ASSOCIATION AND ACADEMY OF HEALTH INFORMATION PROFESSIONALS

Closer to home is an array of library associations and organizations related to the health sciences. The primary national organization for you is the MLA, which publishes the *Bulletin of the Medical Library Association,* cited throughout this book. The *MLA News* provides updates on association information; legislation affecting health care and libraries; continuing education opportunities; tools of librarianship, including electronic and print sources; annual meeting information; and job openings. Your involvement in MLA may take several paths. There are fourteen regional groups (e.g., the South Central chapter is composed of Arkansas, Louisiana, New Mexico, Oklahoma, and Texas). These regional chapters as well as state associations of medical librarians also have meetings and supply continuing education activities. The health sciences librarian may also be active in various subject interest sections of MLA, such as the following:

—Cancer Librarians

—Chiropractic Libraries

—Collection Development

—Consumer and Patient Health Information

—Dental

—Educational Media and Technologies

—Federal Libraries

—History of Health Sciences

—Hospital Libraries

—International Cooperation

—Library Research

—Medical Informatics

—Medical Library Education

—Medical School Libraries

—Medical Society Libraries

—Mental Health Librarians

—Nursing and Allied Health Resources

—Pharmacy and Drug Information

—Public Health/Health Administration Libraries

—Public Services

—Relevant Issues

—Technical Services

—Veterinary Medical Libraries

These groups supply opportunities for librarians to work together, to educate each other, and to advance the interests of the field. For many years the MLA has had a certification program. In 1989 MLA changed from an examination to a portfolio system of certification. The program's new title is Academy of Health Information Professionals. To qualify an applicant needs to show mastery of ten subject areas as well as experience in the field. An MLA task force on knowledge and skills arrived at an array of competencies a health sciences librarian needs and determined that the ten following areas are critical:

Health Care Environment

Medical Concepts and Terminology

Information Needs of Health Professionals

Computer Hardware, Software, and Information-Related Applications

Basic Research Techniques

Basic Management Principles

Acquiring and Organizing Information

MeSH and NLM Classification

Information Sources in the Health Sciences

Online Searching (including MEDLINE)

This book is intended to get you started in several of these. Along with mastering the basics, you are expected to continue your education. This is a key concept. Academy membership lasts five years. During that time you are expected to continue your education by attending conferences and workshops, writing articles, serving professional organizations, and so on. For more on MLA, visit its home page, where you will find information on meetings, text of publications, continuing education opportunities, information policy issues, and employment opportunities. MLANET can currently be found at http://www.kumc.edu/MLA/.

QUALIFICATIONS

The real challenge to us is to grow beyond our traditional roles. MLA's *Platform for Change* comments:

> While information handling was once almost entirely the province of librarians, that is no longer the case. Exponential growth in biomedical knowledge and new information technologies are redefining the infrastructure of health care, education, and research, spawning an array of professional specialties and reworking what was a well-defined arena of information service. (Medical Library Association 1991, 1)

The theme is this: The health care environment is changing. There will be new and great opportunities in the field of health care information. We need to grow and educate ourselves in order to work with the emerging technologies to meet those needs and demands. If we do not grow, others will take up our role.

Since this book is intended for the new health sciences librarian, the first issue of qualifications is this: What do you need to know to become a medical librarian? Traditionally, a liberal arts background has been the foundation for most librarians and that has included medical librarians.You will need also the knowledge and skills the library schools provide—organizing, disseminating, and managing information. But what else? What about the subject requirements? Do you need a degree in science to be a good medical librarian? It would seem helpful. Is it a requirement? Most library schools have a course that delves into the variety of pursuits from which the graduate may choose. The question of educational requirements often comes up. On one of these occasions several years ago, a group of fifteen medical library school students were in attendance with other library school students as different speakers talked about their own libraries and the preparation for their jobs. A pattern emerged from the presentation. Yes, the music librarian said, you really did need that second master's degree in music to pursue the field of music librarianship. The law librarian said that for public service and reference, the J.D. was a requirement. As speaker after speaker finished, the medical library students looked at each other and the question came to their minds: What does this mean for us? What are we supposed to have? An M.D.? Finally, one of them asked that question. The answer came back: No, your courses here in medical librarianship will be just what you need.

This does not really answer the question. It may merely be a reflection of the prevailing reality of supply and demand. Out of that number of fifteen students, only three had science backgrounds. In a 1985 study of the directors of academic health sciences libraries (Anderson 1989), just 19% had health-related degrees. Anecdotal pronouncements can be gathered.

> One factor, that at times I see as dividing the community of medical reference librarians into two vast sectors—the god-like and the great unwashed—is the "science background" bugaboo. In all the reference librarians I've seen or worked with, I've never been able to see any correlation between on-the-job effectiveness and educational background, yet this is a favorite totem I've run into many times since entering library school. (Holohan 1982: 91)

Today, another question might just as likely arise about your qualifications when prospective employers are considering you. What is your computer science background? Have you followed the developments in telecommunications and networks? Perhaps the librarian's best attribute is the ability to solve problems, whether that entails finding why the network or printer is not working or finding answers to questions.

This much seems clear. You will become an expert in the print and electronic literature of the type of library in which you work. If you are in a hospital specializing in obstetrics, you will become expert in the literature on obstetrics; if in a research laboratory focusing on radiation biology, expert in the literature on radiation biology; and so on. At library meetings, the talk is often about the changes needed in librarianship to make sure it plays a prominent role in the progress of the information field. There are warnings that we must become more competent and farsighted with computers and communications technology. If we do not change, it is said, others will take away our traditional role of providing access to information. It is true that new jobs are evolving. Do we have the competencies to do them? Who will become clinical information coordinators? Who will find a way to organize and search the nontraditional information sources? It would be a large mistake to look at this with a defensive posture. It is mandatory for us to acquire new skills. This is exciting; opportunities are there for us. This is what awaits us: the combination of the subject fields of biology, medicine, and health with equally rapidly advancing information technologies. This should enable many more people to get more and better information in a much easier and convenient manner—if we do our jobs. Remember this: Everything does not have to be mastered at once. Find what is useful and apply it. It is reassuring that there is more to learn, and that will enable us to do our jobs better.

OUR JOBS

Functions performed at other types of libraries also need to be done in health sciences libraries. Some differences have been brought out in the related chapters (e.g., Reference). Some positions, however, are unique to health sciences librarianship. Consider the following:

Clinical Medical Librarian. This position is an adaptation of the traditional reference librarian's position. Instead of passively waiting in the library for questions and requests to come in, the clinical medical librarian goes into the hospital, accompanies the medical staff on bedside rounds, and attends conferences of the hospital staff. In this way he or she can directly determine what information is needed. Typically, the librarian will go back to the library, search for the literature, find a few of the most useful articles for the case, and distribute copies to those who need the information. This model of activity should also spread to, and consequently change, the work of the reference librarians.

Circuit Rider Librarian. This position may be very loosely compared to that of a librarian who works from a bookmobile. Library services are brought to those who are isolated from good medical collections and services. There are hospitals that are too small to support a full-time librarian, for example. In cooperation with a large medical library, usually a medical school library, a few hospitals arrange to have a librarian come to each of them periodically. The circuit rider librarian gathers the requests from the hospital personnel and also spends time at the larger library to retrieve the information that has been requested. With fax machines, modems, and the Internet, this service can also deliver information in a timely manner.

Personal Information Consultant. This individual assists health care professionals and researchers organize systems to handle the information they gather and use.

What does make health sciences libraries different? Some positions are unique to the health sciences libraries. Another difference is the patrons, who include physicians, nurses, allied health personnel, and medical students. A third difference is the mission of the patrons: to care for sick people; to investigate the health of sick and healthy people. A fourth difference may be the setting (e.g., a hospital). The information and experience you have from other types of libraries will serve you well. If you have worked in an academic library, keep in mind that many aspects carry over to a medical school library. If you have been running a one-person library, your experience will help you in most hospital libraries. Guy St. Clair (1987) has done quite a bit of writing on the topic of the special library that has only one librarian. Many hospital libraries have a staff of only one librarian or a staff of one librarian and one assistant, and, it is not unusual for a recent graduate of a library school to be hired for that position in a one-person library. Because you are the only one in the whole organization who actually knows what goes on in a library and what needs to be done, you often have a lot of freedom. This does not mean that you have any leisure time and are not hard pressed to get done what needs to be done. However, you can usually decide to do the work in a way that you choose. The traditional library job of cataloging books, for instance, is part of your responsibility. It is your choice how to do it. However, it is also your responsibility to find out that you can obtain most cataloging records electronically for pennies as opposed to creating your own. Because you can do the many library tasks as you determine, there is the danger that you will go on and on in the same way for years. You may work one way because you have always worked that way. It is comfortable. Developments in the library world may offer improvements, but you are the only one in your organization who may know about them. This does not mean that you should adopt every new thing that comes along just because it is new. However, if you are typing catalog cards, for example, and a service is available to get that information electronically at a fraction of the cost, you are not managing your operation in the best interests of anybody—you, your employer, or your patrons. Time is a resource that you need to manage. How should you spend it? How many meetings, for example, can you afford to go to? You need to keep abreast of information in your institution and your field and meetings can help. However, other things need to be attended to as well. In your one-person library, you may not be able to attend library workshops and conferences as often as your academic colleagues. Because only you are keeping tabs on your time, you need to be especially vigilant. You may feel isolated professionally as well as physically from other librarians. A one-person library is not the place for every librarian.

The Janet Doe Lecture on the History or Philosophy of Medical Librarianship is presented each year at the MLA annual meeting. Librarians chosen to give the lecture have had long and distinguished careers in health sciences librarianship. They may speak on almost anything in health sciences librarianship they choose. Ruth Holst (1991), a hospital librarian, gave the 1990 Janet Doe Lecture. She discussed the changing roles of the hospital library in the twentieth century. She concluded with thoughts informally gathered from her colleagues explaining why they like their jobs as hospital librarians. (1) The hospital librarian's job seems to be especially service oriented, and the librarians felt that their contributions are not only used and useful but are also in the pursuit of worthy causes. (2) The environment of the hospital has been less burdened by the hierarchy and bureaucracy found in academic libraries. The librarian can more easily adapt to changes because he or she has the autonomy to act. This is not to say that internal politics are not a prominent consideration in the hospital. However, since there are many people who may have direct input in an academic library, the decision-making process there often drags on for months. (3) The variety of things to do in a hospital library makes it attractive. Also, the medical literature is interesting to many librarians, and this job enables the librarian to work with it more deeply. (4) There are two things about the patrons of our libraries that make for a positive situation. They are typically hard-working and motivated, and we get to know them well over time.

ADAPTING TO THE FUTURE

A lot of attention has been centered here on the hospital and the hospital librarian. Economic forces compel us to make the case of the importance of our service to health care professionals. Even if we are successful in that, the changing environment in health care seems likely to change the institutions in which we have been working. In other words, what happens to us when the hospital, as we know it, no longer exists? Thomas Detre concludes: ''Hospitals, per se, will lose their preeminent role and will be replaced by regional health networks that will integrate outpatient, inpatient, rehabilitation, and home care and incorporate programs aimed at educating patients and their families about the nature of the illness they are dealing with'' (National Library of Medicine 1995d, 3). This NLM report, along with MLA's *Platform for Change*, urges us to develop the skills necessary to work in the new environment. This focuses again on competencies in both technological and management skills. First, we need the skills to handle information of the digital or virtual library. We in librarianship have been discussing this for a long time. We need to continue to expand our competencies in it. Second, we need to create our own roles and alliances with health care professionals. They may be physicians or dentists or nurse practitioners. However, they may not be situated in the one place where we physically work. In order for us to continue in our role, librarians need to show health care professionals that they as individual providers or groups of providers need us as the way to obtain efficiently the information they need. This will require more than our technological know how. This may call for our becoming information entrepreneurs and running our service without the umbrella of something like a hospital to cover us. In our immediate future, medical schools are attempting to move away from the regimen of memorization to problem-based learning (Schilling et al. 1995). This takes students away from their textbooks and into challenging them to use the larger world of information. This provides the incentive for students and the opportunities for us. We should find and take the initiative in involving ourselves in nursing education (Layton and Hahn 1995). We must, as well, seek others in need of information in the health sciences.

OUR SERVICE

A few comments on qualifications relating to education and experience have been put forward. Something needs to be mentioned about the personal attributes of the health sciences librarian. The quality of the library is measured by the service it provides its patrons. The librarian makes the difference. Here is a list of desirable characteristics for the librarian: curious, innovative, imaginative, meticulous, dependable. And, of course, you also want the person to be forthright, compassionate, and nice. This list, to which more platitudes could certainly be added, really tells you nothing. What you need to understand is that librarians can turn their services into as much or little as they choose. A real obstacle to service can be the librarian. When confronted with a new situation, some librarians think first of the reasons why they or the library cannot or should not be involved in it. Perhaps the overriding virtue is this: You need to be the type of person who looks at a problem and thinks first about ways to address it. You should understand that, in reality, you often have a broader license than you assume. Be creative and innovative. There are many opportunities for us.

The goal of the health sciences is to improve the health of people and to provide the best possible health care. The level of care is dependent on the state of knowledge. If our service is to provide that information, how can we get a clear picture of how our contribution helps? It is usually difficult to trace an improvement in an individual's health back to one piece of information a physician received. However, sometimes it can be done. A letter to the *New England Journal of Medicine* provides an example (Sohn and Robbins 1985). While operating, a surgeon encountered a large mass. A biopsy was done, but the surgeon was not sure what procedure should be followed. Still during the operation, a computer search of the medical literature was done on MEDLINE. From the literature it was determined that removal of the mass was not indicated and that drug therapy would be effective. You may be thinking: "I certainly would not want this doctor as my surgeon. I want someone who knows what he or she is doing." That is not an uncommon or surprising reaction. However, is not an open mind and a willingness to learn what you really want? Do we, too, just give that lip service, or do we really mean it? Hopefully, we are not clinging to the notion of the all-knowing physician. Health care providers need information. We know how to find the information they need. Admittedly, not many cases show the role of information provision as dramatically as this case.

Whether the library is digital or virtual or even print on paper, for the best testimonial, look at the well-known comments of William Osler. At the beginning of the twentieth century, he had some things to say about our role: "It is hard for me to speak of the value of libraries in terms which would not seem exaggerated" (Osler 1904, 220). And he continues:

> For the general practitioner a well-used library is one of the few correctives of the premature senility which is so apt to overtake him. Self-centred, self-taught, he leads a

solitary life, and unless his every-day experience is controlled by careful reading or by the attrition of a medical society it soon ceases to be of the slightest value and becomes a mere accretion of isolated facts, without correlation. It is astonishing with how little reading a doctor can practise medicine, but it is not astonishing how badly he may do it. (Osler 1904, 221)

Bibliography

Adams, Scott. 1972. The way of the innovator: Notes toward a prehistory of MEDLARS. *Bulletin of the Medical Library Association* 60, no. 4 (October):523–533.

Adams, Scott. 1981. *Medical bibliography in an age of discontinuity*. Chicago: Medical Library Association.

Almagro, Bertha R. 1984. Book reviewing in medical journals. *Serials Librarian* 9, no. 2 (Winter):121–131.

Altman, Lawrence K. 1995. Revisionist history sees Pasteur as liar who stole rival's ideas. *New York Times* 144 (May 16):C1, C3.

Altschul, Stephen F. et al. 1990. Basic local alignment search tool. *Journal of Molecular Biology* 215, no. 3 (October 5):403–410.

American Hospital Association. 1991. *Survey of health sciences libraries in hospitals, 1989: Executive summary*. Chicago: American Hospital Association.

American Hospital Association. 1993. *Hospital statistics*, 1993–94 ed. Chicago: American Hospital Association.

American Medical Association. 1995. *Drug evaluations annual, 1995*. Chicago: American Medical Association.

American Psychological Association. 1992. *PsycINFO user manual*. Washington, DC: American Psychological Association.

Anderson, Rachael K. 1989. Reinventing the medical librarian. *Bulletin of the Medical Library Association* 77, no. 4 (October):323–331.

Angell, Marcia and Kassirer, Jerome P. 1991. The Ingelfinger Rule revisited. *New England Journal of Medicine* 325, no. 19 (November 7):1371–1373.

Association of American Medical Colleges. 1984. *Physicians for the twenty-first century: The GPEP Report*. Washington, DC: Association of American Medical Colleges.

Barnett, G. Octo; Jenders, Robert A.; and Chueh, Henry C. 1993. The computer-based clinical record—Where do we stand? *Annals of Internal Medicine* 119, no. 10 (November 15):1046–1048.

Bartlett, John. 1980. *Familiar quotations*, 15th ed., ed. E. M. Beck. Boston: Little, Brown.

Bennett, Howard J. 1992. Keeping up with the literature. *JAMA* 267, no. 7 (February 19):920.

Berner, Eta S. et al. 1994. Performance of four computer-based diagnostic systems. *New England Journal of Medicine* 330, no. 25 (June 23):1792–1796.

Berry, Elliot M. 1981. The evolution of scientific and medical journals. *New England Journal of Medicine* 305, no. 7 (August 13):400–402.

Bluh, Pamela. 1993. Document delivery 2000: Will it change the nature of librarianship? *Wilson Library Bulletin* 67, no. 6 (February):49–51, 112.

Bockris, John. 1991. Cold fusion II: The story continues. *New Scientist* 129, no. 1752 (January 19):50–53.

Boyden, Karen, ed. 1994. *Medical and health information directory*, 7th ed. 3 vols. Detroit: Gale Research.

Bradford, Samuel C. 1934. Sources of information on specific subjects. *Engineering* 137 (January 26):85–86.

Bradley, Jana, ed. 1983. *Hospital library management*. Chicago: Medical Library Association.

Brandon, Alfred N. and Hill, Dorothy R. 1992a. Selected list of books and journals in allied health sciences. *Bulletin of the Medical Library Association* 80, no. 3 (July): 223–239.

Brandon, Alfred N. and Hill, Dorothy R. 1992b. Selected list of nursing books and journals. *Nursing & Healthcare* 13, no. 3 (March):139–150.

Brandon, Alfred N. and Hill, Dorothy R. 1993. Selected list of books and journals for the small medical library. *Bulletin of the Medical Library Association* 81, no. 2 (April):141–168.

Brandon, Alfred N. and Hill, Dorothy R. 1994a. Selected list of books and journals in allied health. *Bulletin of the Medical Library Association* 82, no. 3 (July):247–264.

Brandon, Alfred N. and Hill, Dorothy R. 1994b. Selected list of nursing books and journals. *Nursing Outlook* 42, no. 2 (March/April):71–82.

Brandon, Alfred N. and Hill, Dorothy R. 1995. Selected list of books and journals for the small medical library. *Bulletin of the Medical Library Association* 83, no. 2 (April):151–175.

Brandsma, Renze et al. 1990. A comparison of the coverage of clinical medicine provided by BIOSIS Previews and Medline. *Online Review* 14, no. 6 (December):367–377.

Brenner, Saundra H. and McKinin, Emma Jean. 1989. CINAHL and MEDLINE: A comparison of indexing practices. *Bulletin of the Medical Library Association* 77, no. 4 (October):366–371.

Broad, William and Wade, Nicholas. 1982. *Betrayers of the truth*. New York: Simon & Schuster.

Broering, Naomi C. 1993. IAIMS at Georgetown University: The emergence of a high-performance ''virtual library.'' In *High-performance medical libraries: Advances in information management for the virtual era*, ed. N. C. Broering, 7–30. Westport, CT: Meckler.

Brown, Clara D. and Smith, Lynn S. 1980. *Serials: Past, present and future*. Birmingham, AL: EBSCO.

Brownne, John S. 1903. A few hints on medical library administration. *Medical Library and Historical Journal* 1, no. 1 (January):33–34.

Bunting, Alison. 1987. The nation's health information network: History of the Regional Medical Library Program, 1965–1985. *Bulletin of the Medical Library Association* 75, no. 3, supplement (July):1–62.

Bunting, Alison, ed. 1994–. *Current practice in health sciences librarianship*. Metuchen, NJ: Scarecrow Press.

Bunyan, Linda E. and Lutz, Evelyn M. 1991. Marketing the hospital library to nurses. *Bulletin of the Medical Library Association* 79, no. 2 (April):223–225.

Burdick, Amrita J.; Butler, Anne; and Sullivan, Marilyn G. 1993. Citation patterns in the health sciences: Implications for series/monographic fund allocation. *Bulletin of the Medical Library Association* 81, no. 1 (January):44–47.

Carlson, Bob. 1994. Telemedicine changing practice of medicine. *Indiana Medicine* 87, no. 5 (September/October):352–359.

Charen, Thelma. 1983. *MEDLARS indexing manual, pt. 2*. Bethesda, MD: National Library of Medicine.

Charen, Thelma. 1988. Author! author! *NLM Technical Bulletin*, no. 225 (January):14–15.

Clevesy, Sandra and Smith, Bernie Todd. 1993. Finding clinical practice guidelines: Tools for librarians. *National Network* 17, no. 4 (April):20–22.

Cohn, Victor. 1989. *News & numbers: A guide to reporting statistical claims and controversies in health and other fields*. Ames: Iowa State University Press.

Colaianni, Lois Ann. 1991. Letter to MEDLARS network users from the National Library of Medicine. Subject: Clinical trials alert (January 25).

Connelly, Donald P. et al. 1990. Knowledge resource preferences of family physicians. *Journal of Family Practice* 30, no. 3 (March):353–359.

Coronary Artery Surgery Study Group. 1983. Coronary artery surgery study (CASS): A randomized trial of coronary artery bypass surgery: Survival data. *Circulation* 68, no. 5 (November):939–950.

Cowley, Geoffrey. 1993. The hunt for a breast cancer gene. *Newsweek* 122, no. 23 (December 6):46–48, 49, 51–52.

Crampon, Jean E. 1988. Murphy, Parkinson, and Peter: Laws for librarians. *Library Journal* 113, no. 17 (October 15):37–41.

Cummings, Martin M. and Corning, Mary E. 1971. The Medical Library Assistance Act: An analysis of the NLM extramural programs, 1965–1970. *Bulletin of the Medical Library Association* 59, no. 3 (July):375–391.

Dalrymple, Prudence W., ed. 1993. Libraries and information services in the health sciences. *Library Trends* 42, no. 1 (summer):1–223.

Darling, Louise, ed. 1982–1988. *Handbook of medical library practice*. 4th ed. 3 vols. Chicago: Medical Library Association.

Davies, Nicholas E. 1982. Do hospitals need libraries? *Annals of Internal Medicine* 97, no. 6 (December):924–925.

Dick, Richard S. and Steen, Elaine B., eds. 1991. *The computer-based patient record: An essential technology for health care*. Washington, DC: National Academy Press.

Dupree, A. Hunter. 1957. *Science in the federal government: A history of policies and activities to 1940*. Cambridge, MA: Belknap Press.

Durack, David T. 1978. The weight of medical knowledge. *New England Journal of Medicine* 298, no. 14 (April 6):773–775.

Elmer-DeWitt, Philip. 1994. The genetic revolution. *Time* 143, no. 3 (January 17):46–53.

Fenske, Ruth E. and Fortney, Lynn M. 1986. A glossary of medical library jargon. *Medical Reference Services Quarterly* 5, no. 2 (summer):45–75.

Flannery, Melinda Reagor. 1995. Cataloging Internet resources. *Bulletin of the Medical Library Association* 83, no. 2 (April):211–215.

Flexner, Abraham. 1910. *Medical education in the United States and Canada: A report to the Carnegie Foundation for the Advancement of Teaching*. New York: Arno Press.

Fortney, Lynn M. and Basile, Victor A. 1995. *Index Medicus price study*. Birmingham, AL: EBSCO.

Fredericksen, Richard B. and Michael, Helen N. 1976. Subject cataloging practices in North American medical school libraries. *Bulletin of the Medical Library Association* 64, no. 4 (October):356–366.

Friede, Andrew; Reid, Joseph A.; and Ory, Howard W. 1993. CDC—WONDER: A comprehensive on-line public health information system of the Centers for Disease Control and Prevention. *American Journal of Public Health* 83, no. 9 (September):1289–1294.

Friedman, Emily. 1990. Troubled past of ''invisible'' profession. *JAMA* 264, no. 22 (December 12):2851–2852, 2854–2855, 2858.

Funk, Mark E. and Reid, Carolyn Anne. 1983. Indexing consistency in MEDLINE. *Bulletin of the Medical Library Association* 71, no. 2 (April):176–183.

Fye, W. Bruce. 1987. The literature of American internal medicine: A historical view. *Annals of Internal Medicine* 106, no. 3 (March):451–460.

Gable, Carol Brignoli. 1990. A compendium of public health data sources. *American Journal of Epidemiology* 131, no. 3 (March):381–394.

Garfield, Eugene, ed. 1989. *SCI journal citation reports: A bibliometric analysis of science journals in the ISI data base*. Philadelphia: Institute for Scientific Information.

Ginzberg, Eli. 1983. Allied health resources. In *Handbook of health, health care, and the health professions*, ed. D. Mechanic, 479–494. New York: Free Press.

Ginzberg, Eli and Dutka, Anna B. 1989. *The financing of biomedical research*. Baltimore: Johns Hopkins University Press.

Glowniak, Jerry V. and Bushway, Marilyn K. 1994. Computer networks as a medical resource: Accessing and using the Internet. *JAMA* 271, no. 24 (June 22–29):1934–1939.

Goddard, Catherine F. 1993. Online sources of health sciences book reviews. *Medical Reference Services Quarterly* 12, no. 4 (Winter):23–36.

Gonick, Larry and Wheelis, Mark. 1991. *The cartoon guide to genetics*. Updated ed. New York: HarperPerennial.

Gorry, G. Anthony. 1992. IAIMS development at Baylor College of Medicine. *Bulletin of the Medical Library Association* 80, no. 3 (July):247–252.

Gradler, Geoffrey C. and Schrammel, Kurt E. 1994. The 1992–2005 job outlook in brief. *Occupational Outlook Quarterly* 38, no. 1 (Spring):2–45.

Greenes, Robert A. and Shortliffe, Edward H. 1990. Medical informatics: An emerging academic discipline and institutional priority. *JAMA* 263, no. 8 (February 23): 1114–1120.

Gregor, Dorothy and Mandel, Carol. 1991. Cataloging must change! *Library Journal* 116, no. 6 (April):42–47.

Guarding the guardians: Research on editorial peer review; international congress, 1st. 1990. *JAMA* 263, no. 10 (March 9):1317–1441.

Guterman, Stuart et al. 1988. The first 3 years of Medicare prospective payment: An overview. *Health Care Financing Review* 9, no. 3 (spring):67–77.

Hancock, Lee. 1994. CancerNet: More than PDQ on the Net. *Database* 17, no. 1 (February):86–88.

Harvard guidelines for investigators in scientific research. 1989. *Clinical Research* 37, no. 2 (April):192–193.

Haynes, R. Brian. 1990. Loose connections between peer-reviewed clinical journals and clinical practice. *Annals of Internal Medicine* 113, no. 9 (November 1):724–728.

Haynes, R. Brian et al. 1986. How to keep up with the medical literature: I. Why try to keep up and how to get started. *Annals of Internal Medicine* 105, no. 1 (July): 149–153.

Hickey, Thomas B. 1995. Present and future capabilities of the online journal. *Library Trends* 43, no. 4 (spring): 528–543.

Hill, Lister. 1966. The medical library crisis: Billings to MEDLARS. *Journal of Medical Education* 41, no. 1 (January):80–84.

Holohan, John S. 1982. 10,000 days on the reference desk. *Medical Reference Services Quarterly* 1, no. 1 (spring):89–93.

Holst, Ruth. 1991. Hospital libraries in perspective. *Bulletin of the Medical Library Association* 79, no. 1 (January):1–9.

Humphrey, Susanne M. 1989. MedIndEx system: Medical indexing expert system. *Information Processing & Management* 25, no. 1:73–88.

Hunter, Janne A. 1991. MEDLINE on BRS, Data-Star and DIALOG—Does it make a difference? *Database* 14, no. 1 (February):43–50.

Huth, Edward J. 1989. The underused medical literature. *Annals of Internal Medicine* 110, no. 2 (January 15):99–100.

International congress on peer review in biomedical publication, 2nd. 1994. *JAMA* 272, no. 2 (July 13):91–173.

Jensen, Joseph E. 1981. Hospital libraries: Expensive window dressing or resources for cost-containment? *Maryland State Medical Journal* 30, no. 2 (February):44–45.

Johnson, Nancy R. et al. 1990. The best reference books in a medical school library: What your colleagues say. *Medical Reference Services Quarterly* 9, no. 4 (Winter):43–79.

Kassirer, Jerome P. and Angell, Marcia. 1995. The Internet and the Journal. *New England Journal of Medicine* 332, no. 25 (June 22):1709–1710.

Keleher, Cynthia. 1993. Translating the genetic library: The goals, methods, and applications of the Human Genome Project. *Bulletin of the Medical Library Association* 81, no. 3 (July):274–277.

Ketcham, Lee and Born, Kathleen. 1995. Serials vs. the dollar dilemma: Currency swings and rising costs play havoc with prices. *Library Journal* 120, no. 7 (April 15): 43–49.

King, David N. 1987. The contribution of hospital library information services to clinical care: A study in eight hospitals. *Bulletin of the Medical Library Association* 75, no. 4 (October):291–301.

King, David N. 1989. The service imperative: Do library services improve the quality of patient care? *Bibliotheca Medica Canadiana* 10, no. 3:121–125.

Kingsland III, Lawrence C. et al. 1993. Coach: Applying UMLS Knowledge Sources in an expert searcher environment. *Bulletin of the Medical Library Association* 81, no. 2 (April):178–183.

Klein, Michele S. et al. 1994. Effect of online literature searching on length of stay and patient care costs. *Academic Medicine* 69, no. 6 (June):489–495.

Kroenke, Kurt. 1986. Book reviews in medical journals. *Bulletin of the Medical Library Association* 74, no. 1 (January):1–5.

Kronenfeld, Jennie Jacobs and Whicker, Marcia Lynn. 1984. *U.S. national health policy: An analysis of the federal role.* New York: Praeger.

La Rocco, August. 1994. The role of the medical school–based consumer health information service. *Bulletin of the Medical Library Association* 82, no. 1 (January): 46–51.

Lacroix, Eve-Marie. 1994. Interlibrary loan in U.S. health sciences libraries: Journal article use. *Bulletin of the Medical Library Association* 82, no. 4 (October):363–368.

Lavendel, Giuliana. 1977. Special libraries. *Chemical & Engineering News* 55, no. 16 (April 18):34–42.

Layton, Beth and Hahn, Karla. 1995. The librarian as a partner in nursing education. *Bulletin of the Medical Library Association* 83, no. 4 (October):499–502.

Levine, Fred and Friedmann, Theodore. 1993. Gene therapy. *American Journal of Diseases of Children* 147, no. 11 (November):1167–1174.

Levit, Katharine R. et al. 1994. National health expenditures, 1993. *Health Care Financing Review* 16, no. 1 (Fall):247–294.

Light, Donald W. 1983. Medical and nursing education: Surface behavior and deep structure. In *Handbook of health, health care, and the health professions*, ed. D. Mechanic, 455–478. New York: Free Press.

Lindberg, Donald A. B. et al. 1993. Use of MEDLINE by physicians for clinical problem solving. *JAMA* 269, no. 24 (June 23–30):3124–3129.

Lorenzi, Nancy M., ed. 1992. Symposium: A decade of IAIMS. *Bulletin of the Medical Library Association* 80, no. 3 (July):240–293.

Lucky, Robert W. 1989. *Silicon dreams: Information, man, and machine*. New York: St. Martin's Press.

Maher, John. 1986. The development of English as an international language of medicine. *Applied Linguistics* 7, no. 2:206–218.

Marshall, Eliot. 1994. NIH tunes up peer review. *Science* 263, no. 5151 (March 4):1212–1213.

Marshall, Joanne G. 1992. The impact of the hospital library on clinical decision making: The Rochester study. *Bulletin of the Medical Library Association* 80, no. 2 (April):169–178.

Martin, Nadia J.; Primich, Tracy; and Riley, Ruth A. 1994. Accessing genetics databases. *Database* 17, no. 1 (February):51–58.

Marwick, Charles. 1990. How do they conduct "N-HANES," anyway? *JAMA* 263, no. 19 (May 16):2581.

Matassarin-Jacobs, Esther. 1989. The nursing licensure process and the NCLEX-RN. *Nurse Educator* 14, no. 6 (November/December):32–35.

Matheson, Nina W. and Cooper, John A. D. 1982. Academic information in the academic health sciences center: Roles for the library in information management. *Journal of Medical Education* 57, no. 10, pt. 2 (October):1–93.

Mazza, Joseph J. 1994. A library for internists. VIII. Recommendations from the American College of Physicians. *Annals of Internal Medicine* 120, no. 8 (April 15): 699–720.

McDonald, Kim A. 1995. Too many co-authors? *Chronicle of Higher Education* 41, no. 33 (April 28):A35–A36.

Medical Library Association. 1991. *Platform for change: The educational policy statement of the Medical Library Association.* Chicago: Medical Library Association.

Medical Library Association. 1994. *Standards for hospital libraries.* Chicago: Medical Library Association.

Medical Library Association. 1995. *Directory of the Medical Library Association, 1995/96.* Chicago: Medical Library Association.

Mehnert, Robert. 1995. National Library of Medicine. In *The Bowker annual library and book trade almanac*, 165–171. New York: Bowker.

Miles, Wyndham D. 1982. *A history of the National Library of Medicine, the nation's treasury of medical knowledge.* Bethesda, MD: National Library of Medicine.

Muench, Eugene V. 1979. *Biomedical subject headings: A reconciliation of National Library of Medicine (MeSH) and Library of Congress subject headings.* 2nd ed. Hamden, CT: Shoe String Press.

National Library of Medicine. 1985. *Collection development manual of the National Library of Medicine.* Bethesda, MD: National Library of Medicine.

National Library of Medicine. 1993a. 3,000,000 characters a day. *Gratefully Yours* (May/June):4.

National Library of Medicine. 1993b. *Collection development manual of the National Library of Medicine.* 3rd ed. Bethesda, MD: National Library of Medicine.

National Library of Medicine. 1993c. *Fact sheet: Online indexing system.* Bethesda, MD: National Library of Medicine.

National Library of Medicine. 1994a. Cataloging practices. In *Medical subject headings—annotated alphabetic list, 1995.* Bethesda, MD: National Library of Medicine, I-145–I-178.

National Library of Medicine. 1994b. Publication types, 1995. In *Medical subject headings—annotated alphabetic list, 1995.* Bethesda, MD: National Library of Medicine, I-18–I-26.

National Library of Medicine. 1995a. *Fact sheet: National Library of Medicine.* Bethesda, MD: National Library of Medicine.

National Library of Medicine. 1995b. ELHILL 3.4: Proximity searching. *NLM Technical Bulletin*, no. 282 (January-February):1, 8–16.

National Library of Medicine. 1995c. *Fact sheet: The visible human project.* Bethesda, MD: National Library of Medicine.

National Library of Medicine. 1995d. *The education and training of health sciences librarians.* Bethesda, MD: National Library of Medicine.

National Library of Medicine. 1995e. Introduction. *Index Medicus* 36, no. 5, pt. 1 (May): viii–xi.

National Library of Medicine. Board of Regents. 1989. *Improving health professionals' access to information*. Bethesda, MD: National Institutes of Health.

Osler, William. 1904. *Aequanimitas*. Philadelphia: P. Blakiston's Sons & Co.

Oxman, Andrew D.; Sackett, David L.; and Guyatt, Gordon H. 1993. Users' guides to the medical literature: How to get started. *JAMA* 270, no. 17 (November 3):2093–2097.

Palmore, James A. and Gardner, Robert W. 1983. *Measuring mortality, fertility, and natural increase: A self-teaching guide to elementary measures*. Honolulu: East-West Center.

Pizer, Irwin H. 1984. Looking backward, 1984–1959: Twenty-five years of library automation—a personal view. *Bulletin of the Medical Library Association* 72, no. 4 (October):335–348.

Poyer, Robert K. 1984. Journal article overlap among *Index Medicus*, *Science Citation Index*, *Biological Abstracts*, and *Chemical Abstracts*. *Bulletin of the Medical Library Association* 72, no. 4 (October):353–357.

Preschel, Barbara M. 1989. Indexing for print, online, and CD-ROM. In *Indexing: The state of our knowledge and the state of our ignorance*, ed. B. H. Weinberg, 52–59. Medford, NJ: Learned Information.

Price, Derek J. de Solla. 1986. *Little science, big science . . . and beyond*. New York: Columbia University Press.

Pritchard-Schoh, Teresa. 1993. Natural language comes of age. *Online* 17, no. 3 (May): 33–43.

Putney, Taylor and Roper, Fred W. 1994. Terminology. In *Introduction to reference sources in the health sciences*, ed. F. W. Roper and J. A. Boorkman, 121–134. Metuchen, NJ: Scarecrow Press.

The quality march. 1993. *Hospitals & Health Networks* 67, no. 23 (December 5):52, 54–55.

Quinn, Judy and Rogers, Michael. 1992. Serials librarians form Aqueduct Action Group. *Library Journal* 117, no. 9 (May 15):12–13.

Rada, Roy et al. 1992. The GALEN dream: *International Classification* 19, no. 4:188–191.

Relman, Arnold. 1981. Journals. In *Coping with the biomedical literature*, ed. D. Kronick, 67–78. New York: Praeger.

Reverby, Susan M. 1987. *Ordered to care: The dilemma of American nursing, 1850–1945*. New York: Cambridge University Press.

Riesenberg, Don and Lundberg, George D. 1990. The order of authorship: Who's on first? *JAMA* 264, no. 14 (October 10):1857.

Roderer, Nancy K. and Clayton, Paul D. 1992. IAIMS at Columbia-Presbyterian Medical Center: Accomplishments and challenges. *Bulletin of the Medical Library Association* 80, no. 3 (July):253–262.

Rogers, Frank B. 1961. Preface. In *Index-catalogue of the library of the Surgeon General's Office*, III. Washington, DC: U.S. Government Printing Office.

Roper, Fred W. and Boorkman, Jo Anne. 1994. *Introduction to reference sources in the health sciences*. 3rd ed. Metuchen, NJ: Scarecrow Press.

Rosenthal, Nadia. 1994. DNA and the genetic code. *New England Journal of Medicine* 331, no. 1 (July 7):39–41.

Rosenzweig, Robert M. 1991. The debate over indirect costs raises fundamental policy issues. *Chronicle of Higher Education* 37 (March 6):A40.

St. Clair, Guy. 1987. The one-person library: An essay on essentials revisited. *Special Libraries* 78, no. 4 (Fall):263–270.

Scheerer, George and Hines, Lois E. 1974. Classification systems used in medical libraries. *Bulletin of the Medical Library Association* 62, no. 3 (July):273–280.

Schilling, Katherine et al. 1995. Integration of information-seeking skills and activities into a problem-based curriculum. *Bulletin of the Medical Library Association* 83, no. 2 (April):176–183.

Schmidt, Karen A, ed. 1990. *Understanding the business of library acquisitions*. Chicago: American Library Association.

Schroeder, Steven A.; Zones, Jane S.; and Showstack, Jonathan A. 1989. Academic medicine as a public trust. *JAMA* 262, no. 6 (August 11):803–812.

Sewell, Winifred. 1964. Medical subject headings in MEDLARS. *Bulletin of the Medical Library Association* 52, no. 1 (January):164–170.

Shortell, Stephen M. 1991. *Effective hospital-physician relationships*. Ann Arbor, MI: Health Administration Press Perspectives.

Shortliffe, Edward H. and Perreault, Leslie E, eds. 1990. *Medical informatics, computer applications in health care*. Reading, MA: Addison-Wesley Publishing.

Smith, Genevieve L. and David, Phyllis E. 1991. *Medical terminology: A programmed text*. 6th ed. Albany, NY: Delmar.

Snow, Bonnie. 1989. Review articles in MEDLINE: Past and present. *Online* 13, no. 2 (March):101–105.

Snow, Bonnie. 1993. Full-text healthcare business sources online. *Online* 17, no. 2 (March):103–108.

Sohn, Norman and Robbins, Richard D. 1985. Computer-assisted surgery. *New England Journal of Medicine* 312, no. 14 (April 4):924.

Spurlock, Sandra and Kovacs, Beatrice. 1986. Selected list of medical journals for the general collection: An annotated bibliography. *Serials Librarian* 11, no. 1 (September):63–106.

Stankus, Tony. 1987. *Scientific journals: Issues in library selection and management*. New York: Haworth Press.

Stankus, Tony. 1992. *Making sense of journals in the life sciences: From specialty origins to contemporary assortment*. New York: Haworth Press.

Stein, Leonard I.; Watts, David T.; and Howell, Timothy. 1990. The doctor-nurse game revisited. *New England Journal of Medicine* 322, no. 8 (February 22):546–549.

Strickland, Stephen P. 1989. *The story of the NIH grants programs*. New York: University Press of America.

Swanson, Don R. 1986. Undiscovered public knowledge. *Library Quarterly* 56, no. 2 (April):103–118.

Tenopir, Carol. 1994. Target, Freestyle, WIN . . . searching takes on a new look. *Library Journal* 119, no. 4 (March 1):34, 36.

Tilley, Carolyn B. 1990. Medical databases and health information systems. *Annual Review of Information Science and Technology* 25:313–382.

Title change hall of fame. 1974. *Title Varies* 1, no. 6 (November):40.

Truelson, Stanley D. 1976. Selecting for health sciences library collections when budgets falter. *Bulletin of the Medical Library Association* 64, no. 2 (April):187–195.

Tuttle, Marcia, ed. *The Newsletter on Serials Pricing Issues [electronic bulletin board]*. available from listserv@gibbs.oit.unc.edu.

United States. President's Commission on Heart Disease, Cancer and Stroke. 1964–65.

A national program to conquer heart disease, cancer and stroke. 2 vols. Washington, DC.

Veatch, Robert M. 1986. DRGs and the ethical reallocation of resources. *Hastings Center Report* 16, no. 3 (June):32–40.

Walsh, Jim and Bothmer, A. James, compilers. 1991. *Vital and health statistics series: An annotated checklist and index to the publications of the "Rainbow series."* Westport, CT: Greenwood Press.

Waserman, Manfred J. 1972. Historical chronology and selected bibliography relating to the National Library of Medicine. *Bulletin of the Medical Library Association* 60, no. 4 (October):551–558.

Washington University (St. Louis) Medical School Library. 1993. Tables on subscription costs. *Newsletter* (Fall):11–14.

Weatherall, David. 1995. *Science and the quiet art: The role of medical research in health care.* New York: W. W. Norton.

Williamson, John W. et al. 1989. Health sciences information management and continuing education of physicians: A survey of U.S. primary care practitioners and their opinion leaders. *Annals of Internal Medicine* 110, no. 2 (January 15):151–160.

Wilson, Mark C. et al. 1995. Users' guides to the medical literature. VIII. How to use clinical practice guidelines. B. What are the recommendations and will they help you in caring for your patients? *JAMA* 274, no. 20 (November 22/29):1630–1632.

Witte, Maryls H.; Kerwin, Ann; and Witte, Charles L. 1988. Seminars, clinics, and laboratories on medical ignorance. *Journal of Medical Education* 63, no. 10 (October):793–795.

Woodsmall, Rose Marie and Benson, Dennis A. 1993. Information resources at the National Center for Biotechnology Information. *Bulletin of the Medical Library Association* 81, no. 3 (July):282–284.

Woolf, Patricia K. 1987. Ensuring integrity in biomedical publication. *JAMA* 258, no. 23 (December 18):3424–3427.

Index

About the Author

FRANK R. KELLERMAN is Biomedical Reference/Collection Development Librarian at Brown University and an Instructor in the Graduate School of Library and Information Studies at the University of Rhode Island. His articles have appeared in journals such as *Science and Technology Libraries* and *RQ*.